Advances in Child Neuropsychology

Advances in
Child Neuropsychology

Edited by

Michael G. Tramontana
Stephen R. Hooper

Michael G. Tramontana
Stephen R. Hooper

Editors

Advances in Child Neuropsychology

Volume 3

With 39 Illustrations

Springer-Verlag
New York Berlin Heidelberg London Paris
Tokyo Hong Kong Barcelona Budapest

Michael G. Tramontana, Ph.D.
Division of Child and Adolescent Psychiatry
Vanderbilt University School of Medicine
Nashville, TN 37212, USA

Stephen R. Hooper, Ph.D.
Department of Psychiatry and the Clinical Center for the Study of Development and Learning
University of North Carolina School of Medicine
Chapel Hill, NC 27514, USA

ISSN: 0940-8606

Printed on acid-free paper.

Production coordinated by Chernow Editorial Services, Inc., and managed by Francine McNeill; manufacturing supervised by Jacqui Ashri.
Typeset by Best-set Typesetter Ltd., Hong Kong.
Printed and bound by Braun-Brumfield, Inc., Ann Arbor, MI.
Printed in the United States of America.

9 8 7 6 5 4 3 2 1

ISBN 0-387-94302-1 Springer-Verlag New York Berlin Heidelberg
ISBN 3-540-94302-1 Springer-Verlag Berlin Heidelberg New York

To Maryanne and our precious gifts—
Michael, Christopher, and Joseph.

M.G.T.

To Mary with much love. Thank you
for your patience, support, and understanding.

S.R.H.

Foreword

In this, the third volume of *Advances in Child Neuropsychology*, the editors have once again enlisted a broad range of contributors, each of whom has written a chapter that brings us to the current level of knowledge in their respective area. The topics range from the relationship between electrophysiological responses in infants and later language development to advances in neuropsychological constructs. Although we still do not know enough about brain–behavior relationships in the normally developing brain, let alone in the atypical brain, a good deal of innovative, exciting, and very meaningful research is herein presented that furthers our understanding of neurodevelopmental issues. The current volume reflects some of the results of an active period of research in child neuropsychology. It serves to further our knowledge of the field in all of its diversity and, perhaps, to provide the spark of interest or sudden "aha!" to the reader that will lead to new insights and productive research endeavors.

The first chapter, contributed by Molfese, is perhaps somewhat technical in its presentation for the electrophysiologically uninitiated. However, its results and discussion sections follow up findings related to some of the data presented in Volume 1. The earlier work, which suggested that electrophysiological responses can be used to predict long-term developmental outcomes, is supported in the present report on the relationship between auditory evoked responses in infancy and later levels of language development. In addition to shedding light on the neurophysiological substrates of early language development, these studies offer promise for the development of valuable tools in the identification of a prevalent developmental disability, developmental language disorders with specifiable cognitive sequela, reading disabilities among them.

In Chapter 2, Bellinger, writing from a public health/neurocognitive point of view, presents a cogent review of the recent literature related to lead exposure and neurocognitive function in children. The review sets the stage for a presentation of data resulting from a multisite, prospective study, elegant in its careful consideration of a complex web of variables. The results suggest that, although lead load and neurocognitive function may be related, many other variables must be taken into account as one interprets research findings. He also points out that no specifiable pattern of neuropsychological dysfunction serves as a "fingerprint" for lead exposure. As important as the results are, Bellinger reflects on the need for neuropsychologists who followed children exposed to a variety of neurotoxins, of which lead is only one example, to develop a "greater appreciation of concepts and methods that generally do not arise in the neuropsychological study of other medical conditions and events." He includes for consideration such factors as toxicokinetics, lead/socio-demographic variables, and the effects of lead exposure on the development of the central nervous system. In all, a thought-provoking chapter.

Bigler, in Chapter 3, makes the case for merging quantitative neuro-imaging and neuropsychological findings, and presents data that represent the beginnings of such an integration. He also reviews the seminal literature on relationships between neuroimaging studies and specific neuro-logic, developmental, and psychiatric disorders. Bigler discusses and applauds the movement toward the quantification of neuroanatomic structures, normal and abnormal, while emphasizing the need for continued qualitative description of brain structures as elucidated by neuro-imaging techniques. The quest, a methodology that will permit the integration of quantitative neuropsychological and neuroimaging data, is pursued, for example, in the specific case material in which both sets of data representing specific patients are given. Although in its infancy, the approach, as discussed by Bigler, appears to be viable and presents exciting prospects.

The NEPSY, a test under development by Korkman and colleagues, is the focus of Chapter 4. Korkman presents a brief overview of approaches to assessment, and describes the rationale for the NEPSY as a set of measures for use in the neuropsychological evaluation of children. Much of the chapter is devoted to the description of the domains and subtests included in the NEPSY, indicating its strong points (e.g., the simultaneous standardization of a goodly number of measures on the same group) and its deficiencies (e.g., lack of a theoretical base). Three studies are presented—two already in the literature, one in press—that demonstrate predictive validity of some of the subtests, discriminative validity of the NEPSY when applied to two clinical groups, and the use of the NEPSY in a follow-up paradigm. In addition, the clinical application of the instrument is demonstrated in a detailed case study. Korkman takes the position that such an instrument would add a great deal to the assessment armamentarium for use with young children. It is certainly the case that the present armamentarium could use some beefing up!

Forster and Leckliter, in Chapter 5, presented an informed discussion of the construct validity of three widely used assessment instruments, the

Halstead-Reitan Neuropsychological Test Battery for Older Children (HRB-OC), the Wide-Range Assessment of Memory and Learning (WRAML), and the Wechsler Intelligence Scale for Children—Third Edition (WISC-III), within the framework of "working memory." To do so, they offer detailed metaanalysis of factor analytic studies involving the three assessment instruments. The authors point out that the model of memory is shifting from one of capacity (short-term memory) to one of process (working memory and executive functions), and that this shift is being reflected in the increasing numbers of papers that have addressed working memory and executive functions in children. They suggest that this shift is being reflected in test development, for example in the WRAML, the most recent of the three, in which working memory is explicitly assessed in a variety of ways. They note that there is increasing appreciation and understanding of the way in which standardized measures assess working memory, leading to more appropriate interpretation of assessment data. Further, Forster and Leckliter have proposed possible relationships between working memory and executive functions, and existing constructs such as "Freedom from Distractibility." They see these theoretical and research challenges leading toward an integrated theoretical framework for child neuropsychology. This is a thoughtful and timely contribution to the volume.

The concluding chapter, contributed by Bakker and colleagues, is a capsule capitulation of the way in which neuropsychology proceeds: the formulation of a problem in brain–behavior terms, the development of a theory-driven model from which experiments are generated, and in the case of child neuropsychology, to include within it a developmental focus, the elaboration of the model as data dictate, a search for congruent validation of the model, and where appropriate and feasible, the application of research findings, buttressed by a viable model, to clinical settings. Bakker has taken such a route. An initial set of hypotheses has, over the past dozen or so years, led to theory and model building, an ongoing series of studies that have ramifications for brain–behavior relationships well beyond the reading process and the development of experimental intervention techniques.

More specifically, the chapter provides a brief but well-synthesized description of Bakker's Balance Model of the reading process, a description of his earlier studies, and a focused literature review that will be useful to anyone particularly interested in this area. Bakker takes the reader from an understanding of his electrophysiological and behavioral data to an understanding of the rationale for the treatment procedures he and his colleagues have developed.

Bakker is the first to acknowledge that he and his colleagues do not as yet know all they need to know about who should be offered what intervention method; the clinical applications now in progress are presented as methods of assisting some children, which is attested to in the case studies he presents, while continuing to learn about the processes involved in a controlled clinical setting. This is an excellent, eminently readable chapter, providing a paradigm of neuropsychological research.

BARBARA C. WILSON

Preface

Advances in Child Neuropsychology is a multivolume book series designed to serve as a forum for exemplary work and critical information in the rapidly growing field of child neuropsychology. Collectively, the preceding volumes in this series have captured some of the diversity and exciting developments in the field, while also offering fresh insights and raising important questions that could help shape future directions.

This volume continues with the format and organization of Volumes 1 and 2. As before, contributions were sought within four general aspects of neuropsychological work and investigation: developmental neuropsychology, abnormal neuropsychology, assessment, and treatment. The goal was to assure a balanced coverage that includes topics dealing with intervention as well as assessment, and normal as well as abnormal developmental processes. Also, as before, each chapter was organized to provide either (1) an authoritative review of a key substantive area or methodological issue in child neuropsychology, or (2) the exposition of an exemplary line of research or applied work in the field.

Volume 3 consists of six chapters divided into the four general areas noted above. Part I (developmental psychology) is comprised of a chapter by Dennis L. Molfese, in which further findings are presented relating electrophysiological responses in infancy to later language development. This represents an extension of the longitudinal work initially presented in Volume 1 of this series, based now on data from a larger set of children. In Part II (abnormal psychology), David Bellinger provides a thoughtful discussion of current knowledge concerning the neurotoxic effects of lead in children, focusing especially on the pivotal work that he and his colleagues have performed in The Boston Prospective Study. Part III (assessment) covers a variety of topics dealing with advances in the methods of or tools for evaluating brain–behavior relationships. This includes a chapter by Erin D. Bigler, which offers a "state of the art" presentation on the impressive developments in brain imaging techniques. Advances in neuropsychological assessment are then examined from two standpoints. Marit Korkman offers a novel approach, the NEPSY. The chapter by Antonia A. Forster and Ingrid N. Leckliter deals instead with refinements in the construct validity of existing methods, especially as they relate to the evaluation of working memory. In Part IV (treatment), Dirk J. Bakker, Robert Licht, and E. Jan Kappers present a chapter that focuses on the application of hemispheric stimulation techniques in children with dyslexia, an outgrowth of an extensive program of research dealing with the Balance Model of reading and an empirically validated system for classifying subtypes of reading disability. Last, the volume concludes with a brief section offering editorial commentary.

As always, we are grateful to our distinguished group of editorial advisers for their thoughtful input. In alphabetical order, they include Russell Barkley, Raymond Dean, George Hynd, Francis Pirozzolo, Byron Rourke, Michael Rutter, Paul Satz, Otfried Spreen, and Barbara Wilson.

MICHAEL G. TRAMONTANA
STEPHEN R. HOOPER

Contents

IV. Treatment

Contributors

DIRK J. BAKKER, PH.D.
Department of Child Neuropsychology
Free University
Amsterdam, The Netherlands
and
Child Neuropsychological Research Department
Paedological Institute
Amsterdam/Duivendrecht, The Netherlands
and
European Graduate School of Neuropsychology
Amsterdam, The Netherlands

DAVID BELLINGER, PH.D., M.S.
Children's Hospital Boston
Harvard Medical School
and
Neuroepidemiology Unit
Children's Hospital
Boston, MA 02115, USA

ERIN D. BIGLER, PH.D.
Department of Psychology
Brigham Young University
Provo, UT 84602-5543, USA

ANTONIA A. FORSTER, PH.D.
Department of Medical Psychology
The Oregon Health Sciences University
Portland, OR 97201-3098, USA

E. JAN KAPPERS, PH.D.
Out-Patient Clinic and Research Department
for Learning Disabilities
Paedological Institute
Amsterdam/Duivendrecht, The Netherlands

MARIT KORKMAN, PH.D.
Clinic of Child Neurology
and Children's Castle Hospital
Helsinki University
SF-00250 Helsinki, Finland

INGRID N. LECKLITER, PH.D.
Child Development and Rehabilitation Center
The Oregon Health Sciences University
Portland, OR 97201-3098, USA

ROBERT LICHT, PH.D.
Department of Child Neuropsychology
Free University
Amsterdam, The Netherlands
and
Child Neuropsychological Research Department
Paedological Institute
Amsterdam/Duivendrecht, The Netherlands
and
European Graduate School of Neuropsychology
Amsterdam, The Netherlands

DENNIS L. MOLFESE, PH.D.
Department of Psychology
Southern Illinois University
Carbondale, IL 62901, USA

CHAPTER 1

Electrophysiological Responses Obtained During Infancy and Their Relation to Later Language Development: Further Findings

DENNIS L. MOLFESE

In previous reports (Molfese, 1992; Molfese & Molfese, 1993) data were presented strongly supporting the position that early physiological indices could be used to predict long-term developmental outcomes (Molfese & Molfese, 1985). The data in those reports consisted of auditory evoked responses recorded at birth to predict language skills in three-year-old children. Besides finding that later language skills could be predicted from newborn test measures, these longitudinal data were especially striking for the range of the language skills they could differentiate and the time across which they could predict. Although the language skills of the children in the Molfese and Molfese (1985) study covered a considerable range (from relatively poor receptive and productive skills to well-above-average skills), the language skills of the children in the later longitudinal studies (Molfese, 1989, 1992) covered a relatively narrow range of essentially normal language skills. In spite of this similarity reported in the more recent studies, the newborn brain responses continued to effectively distinguish children who performed differently on the language tasks for three years. Molfese (1992) comments, "Consequently, ERPs collected at birth appear to predict with a high degree of accuracy relatively minor differences in language abilities four years later."

These results are further supported by our current longitudinal project, in which data from a larger set of children are now available. In the current study, perinatal, electrophysiological, social, demographic, and environmental variables are all being studied to identify how these variables influence development of cognitive and language skills over the infancy and preschool years. In this chapter we describe the procedures used in the current longitudinal study and reports on the results obtained from analyses exploring the relationship between measures taken in early infancy and subsequent cognitive and language development. To show the similarity between the finding in the current study and our prior studies, the methodology and analysis procedures are identical. The results show that the findings from the current study confirm our prior findings.

Methods

Subjects

In the present report we use a sample of 79 Caucasian children (40 females and 39 males) who were selected from a larger data base of approximately 186 children. These 79 children were selected solely because they had complete data on all the variables being examined here. Most characteristics in this sample are well within the normal range. For example, these children had an average birthweight of 3,406.8 g (SD = 724.3), mean gestational age of 38.2 (SD = 0.45), 1-minute Apgar scores of 7.78 (SD = 1.48), and 5-minute Apgar scores of 8.9 (SD = 0.76). The subjects had a mean Hollinghead two-factor SES score (Bojean, Hill, & McLemore, 1967) of 2.41 (SD = 0.87). Subsequently, all these children were tested on various intelligence tests, including the Stanford-Binet Intelligence Scale (Thorndike, Hagen, & Sattler, 1986). These tests were administered when the children were within two weeks of their third birthday. Although the entire Stanford-Binet Intelligence test was administered, only the results of the Verbal Reasoning subscale are reported here. The mean score on that subscale was 105.4 (SD = 11.3, range = 85–130). The McCarthy Scales of Children's Abilities were also administered (McCarthy, 1972). Their mean score for the McCarthy Verbal Scale Index was 54.6 (SD = 8.68, range = 34–70). In addition, parental responses to the Edinburgh Handedness Inventory (Oldfield, 1971) indicated that each of the parents was strongly right-handed, as indicated by a mean laterality quotient greater than +0.7.

Stimuli

The auditory evoked responses collected were reactions to nine synthetically produced consonant-vowel (CV) syllables. These five-formant synthetic CV syllables, obtained from Dr. Sheila Blumstein, were previously investigated in both behavioral (Blumstein & Stevens, 1980) and electrophysiological studies (Molfese & Schmidt, 1983). The tokens selected for the present study were those most accurately identified by adult participants in the former study as members of their respective categories. These were stimulus tokens 1, 7, and 14 from the /ba, da, ga/ continuum, and tokens 1, 7, and 13 from the /bi, di, gi/ continuum and the /bu, du, gu/ continuum, respectively. These stimuli were originally synthesized on a Klatt cascade synthesizer so that the amplitudes of the individual formants were modulated as a function of the respective formant frequencies, as in natural speech. To further improve the naturalness of the tokens, the vowels /i/ and /u/ were slightly diphthongized. The central frequencies of the steady-state portion of the formants were constant across the different consonant sounds and varied only as a function of the vowels. Duration of the F1 formant transition varied between 15 and 45 ms across the different tokens as a function of the initial consonant sound as well as the following vowel. Transition duration for all other formants was fixed at 40 ms. Voicing duration was 250 ms. Starting frequencies of F2, F3, and F4 were varied systematically across stimuli. Consequently, although starting frequencies for any individual consonant sound varied as a function of the following vowel, the gross shape of the frequency spectrum during the first 25 ms following consonant release remained relatively constant across different vowel contexts. The CV syllables were composed of combinations of three consonants (b, d, g) and three vowels (a, i, u). Two of these CV syllables, /bi, gi/, were similar to two of the syllables that Molfese and Molfese (1985) had found to successfully discriminate low from high language performers, although they did differ from those original tokens in number of formants employed. All the CV syllables were 300 ms in duration, with rise and decay times equated across stimuli. Peak stimulus intensities were also matched. The nine different CVs were arranged on the tape in a block random order, with 20 occurrences of each. The interstimulus interval was varied randomly between 3.5 and 6.0 seconds to reduce habituation and expectancy effects. A square-wave pulse was recorded onto the second channel of the stereo tape and occurred 65 ms before the stimulus on the first channel. This pulse served as a trigger for collecting of the ERPs elicited in response to each stimulus event.

Procedures

As newborns, the subjects were tested within 36 hours of birth using the procedure described here. The head of each infant was first measured to determine where electrodes were to be placed. Six silver-cup scalp electrodes were then placed over the left and right sides of each infant's head. These placements included two electrodes placed respectively over the left (T3) and right (T4) temporal areas of the scalp according to the Ten-Twenty System (Jasper, 1958); a third electrode at FL, a point midway between the external meatus of the left ear and Fz; a fourth electrode at FR, a position midway between the right external meatus and Fz; a fifth electrode at PL, a point midway between the left external meatus and Pz; and a sixth electrode at PR, a point on the right side of the head midway between the right ear's external meatus and Pz. Thus, these electrode placements were over the left frontal (FL), temporal (T3), and parietal (PL) areas of the brain and the corresponding areas of the right hemisphere (FR, T4, and PR, respectively). The electrical activity recorded from all scalp-electrode positions was referred to electrodes placed on each earlobe and linked (A1, A2). Electrode impedances throughout testing were less than 5 kOhm and did not vary more than 1 kOhm between electrode sites on the scalp or the two ear-reference electrodes, as indicated by measurements before and after the test session. It was hoped that such scalp placements would provide information not only on left versus right hemisphere responses, but also general language-perception areas within each hemisphere commonly thought to be localized to the left temporal and parietal language-receptive regions of the brain as well as the language-production areas in the frontal lobe.

Each newborn was tested while in a bed that was reclined at a 40-degree angle throughout the test session. Once the electrodes were placed and the impedances measured, the CV stimuli were presented through a speaker positioned approximately 1 meter over the midline of the infant's head. Stimulus presentation was at 80 dB SPL (A), as measured at the infant's ears, and occurred while the infant was in a quiet awake state. Continuous monitoring of the infant's EEG and EMG and behavioral observation were used to determine when stimulus should be presented. During periods of motor activity, stimulus presentation was suspended. Testing was resumed when the infant's motor activity declined to an acceptable level. The EEG during the test session was amplified 80,000 times with modified Tektronix differential amplifiers with the bandpass flat between 0.1 and 30 Hz. These amplified signals were then recorded onto cassette tape using a Vetter C-8 FM tape recorder. The analogue tapes were then played back offline and the ERP portions of the EEG signal were digitized using a Macintosh Plus microcomputer and the EPACS software package (Molfese, 1988).

For testing at age three years, the parents brought the children to the university laboratory. The children were tested on the Stanford-Binet, including all subtests appropriate for their age and ability. The Stanford-Binet is standardized for use with individuals aged 2 through 23 years. The scale scores can be used to obtain a composite score, as well as subscale scores for Verbal Reasoning, Abstract/Visual Reasoning, Quantitative Reasoning, and Short-Term Memory. Only the Verbal Reasoning scores are reported here. The tests were administered by trained graduate students according to standard procedures.

Analyses

To facilitate comparisons with the work of Molfese and Molfese (1985), the ERP data reduction and initial ERP analysis procedures employed in the earlier study were also applied with this data set. First, 70 data points over a 700-ms period beginning at stimulus onset were digitized for each electrode site, stimulus event, and infant. These digitized values were then stored and subsequent analyses were performed offline following completion of the testing session. Artifact rejection was carried out on the ERP data for each electrode to eliminate from further analyses the ERPs contaminated by motor movements. If an artifact (operationally defined as a shift in voltage level in excess of ± 40 microvolts) occurred on any one electrode channel during the 65-ms pre- or 700-ms poststimulus period, all the ERPs collected across all the electrode sites for that trial were discarded from subsequent analyses. This procedure, based on the peak-to-peak amplitudes of single-trial responses, resulted in rejecting less than 10% of the trials for each infant. Rejection rates were comparable across the nine stimulus conditions. Following artifact rejection, the single-trial data were then averaged separately for each electrode site and stimulus condition. Thus, 54 averages were gathered for each infant. In this manner, 4,266 averaged ERPs were obtained from the 79 infants in response to nine CV syllables, which were composed of three consonants (3: b, d, g), and three vowels (3: a, i, u) from three electrode sites (3: Frontal, Temporal, and Parietal) for each of the two hemispheres (2: Left and Right).

To further facilitate comparisons with the earlier study, the average ERPs recotded in this study were first submitted to a principal-components analysis (PCA) identical to that employed by Molfese and Molfese (1985). This procedure has also been used successfully in previous studies. Although various procedures could be used to analyze the ERP data, this multivariate approach has produced consistent results in programmatic research in a number of laboratories (Brown, Marsh, & Smith, 1979; Chapman, McCrary, Bragdon, & Chapman, 1979; Donchin, Teuting, Ritter, Kutas, & Heffley, 1975; Gelfer, 1987; Molfese, 1978a, 1978b; Molfese & Molfese, 1979, 1980, 1985; Ruchkin, Sutton, Munson, Silver, & Macar, 1981; Segalowitz & Cohen, 1989). For example, Molfese, in papers investigating speech-perception cues such as voice onset time and place of articulation, has found consistent systematic effects across studies for each cue (Molfese, 1978a, 1978b, 1980, 1984; Molfese & Schmidt, 1983). Moreover, these effects have been independently replicated with comparable analysis procedures (Gelfer, 1987; Segalowitz & Cohen, 1989). This procedure is used because it has proven successful both in identifying regions of the ERP where most of the variability occurred across ERPs and subjects, and subsequently in determining if the variability characterized by the different factors was caused by systematic changes in the independent variables being investigated.

The PCA procedure behaves somewhat like a factor analysis, except that it constructs the factors from variances instead of correlations (Rockstroh, Elbert, Birbaumer, & Lutzenberger, 1982, p. 63). The PCA procedure itself is blind to individual experimental conditions and generates the same solution regardless of the order in which the ERPs are entered. Once the PCA identified where within the ERPs most of the variability occurred, a discriminant function procedure used the factor scores generated by the PCA to classify the infants into one of three outcome groups at age 3 that were based on the verbal-performance subtest of the Stanford Binet. This procedure directly addresses the question of whether the newborn ERP waveshapes recorded from different electrode sites over each hemisphere in the region characterized by any one factor could be used to correctly classify these children by their language performance three years later.

Results

The 4,266 averaged auditory evoked responses from the newborn infants each consisted of 70 data points. These data formed the input matrix for the PCA using the BMDP4M program from the BMDP87 package (Dixon, 1986). This program first transformed the data into a covariance matrix and then applied the PCA to this matrix. Seven factors accounting for 88.8% of the variance were selected for further analysis based on the Cattell Scree Test (Cattell, 1966). These factors were then rotated using the normalized varimax criterion (Kaiser, 1958), which preserved the orthogonality among the factors while improving their distinctiveness. This analysis generated factor scores or weights for each of the 4,266 averaged ERPs for each of the seven rotated factors. The variance isolated by the PCA was characterized by the seven factors (factor loadings). The peak for each factor and the area immediately surrounding it in time indicates that this region of the brain wave changed in amplitude or slope across some proportion of the ERPs in the present data.

A factor loading of 0.3 was used for descriptive purposes to identify the region of variability in each of the factors. For the present analyses, only the results from factors 1 and 5 are presented. Factor 1, which accounted for 14.49% of the variance, rose above 0.4 at 140 ms post stimulus onset, reached its maximum value at 240 ms, and dropped below 0.3 at 340 ms post onset. The region of greatest variability for factor 5 began at 570 ms, peaked at 660 ms, and continued to be well above 0.3 at 700 ms.

A factor score was generated by the PCA for each averaged ERP for each factor. Consequently, 4,266 factor scores were generated for factor 1, which reflected the variability across each of the averaged ERPs for the three consonants (3), three vowels (3), six electrode sites (6), and 79 infants; a second set of 4,266 factor scores was generated for factor 2, which identified variability in a different region of the averaged ERPs; a third set of 4,266 factor scores was generated for factor 3, and so on. Only the factor scores from factors 1 and 5, which reflected the amount of variability for that factor in an individual ERP, constituted the dependent variables in the subsequent discriminant-function analysis reported below.

For the discriminant-function procedure, three groups were established with the Stanford-Binet Verbal Reasoning subtest scores obtained for these children at age 3. Of the 79 children, 16 scored at least one SD below the mean, with scores that ranged between 85 and 94; 47 children scored within one SD of the average score of 105.4; and 16 children scored at least one SD above the mean, with scores between 116 and 130.

The two factors in the present analysis that temporally overlapped the two regions of the ERPs previously found by Molfese and Molfese (1985) to discriminate high- from low-language performers were then selected for further analysis. Specifically, in the discriminant-function analysis we used the factor scores from factors 1 and 5, which represented the contributions to the averaged ERP waveforms that were recorded over the six electrode sites in response to the 9 CV syllable stimuli. These factors were then used in an attempt to discriminate at age 3 among the three groups of children: the Low Group, the Mean or average group, and the High group.

The function successfully discriminated 100% of the sample, with 16 children identified as scoring at least one SD below the mean (LOW), 50 children scoring within the average range (AVERAGE), and 13 children scoring at least one SD above the mean (HIGH) for the verbal subtest of the Stanford-Binet. Two discriminant functions were identified that discriminated among the three language groups at age 3. Function 1 accounted for 89.02% of the variance and function 2 accounted for 10.98%. Thus, these two functions together accounted for 100% of the variance for this data set. The chi-square for function 1 was 335.14, with df = 152 and $p < 0.00001$. The canonical correlation for this function was 0.9977. Function 2 had a chi-square of 127.9, with df = 75, $p < 0.0001$. The canonical correlation for this second function was 0.9818.

The group-averaged ERPs from the three groups of infants are depicted in Figure 1.1. The two regions identified by the PCA that overlapped temporally with those reported previously by Molfese and Molfese (1985) are enclosed within the rectangles labeled "1" and "5" for factors 1 and 5, respectively. Notice that the late negative component of the ERP goes markedly negative for the LOW group. The negativity for this region is greatly reduced for the AVERAGE group. For the HIGH group the region generally shows a more flattened appearance before moving upward in a positive direction. In the early portion of the ERP waveform, the duration between the two points labeled "a" and "b" gradually increases as language performance increases. The two points are closest together for the LOW group, at an intermediate point for the AVERAGE group, and more widely separated for the HIGH group.

Discussion

These results indicate that auditory evoked ERPs can successfully discriminate between infants at birth for different levels of language skills as measured by standardized tests three years later. These findings are similar to those previously reported (Molfese & Molfese, 1985). In the previous study, as reviewed earlier, three regions of the ERP waveform discriminated between newborn infants who three years later would

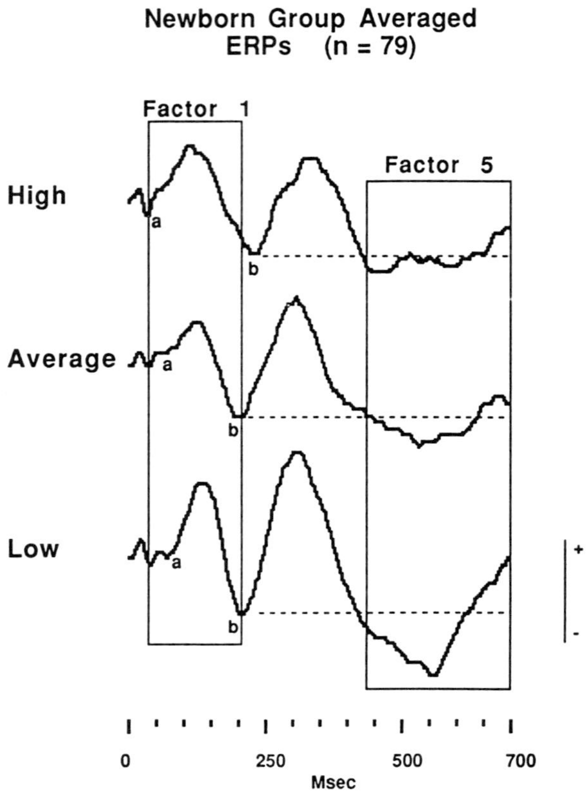

Fig. 1.1. The group-averaged ERPs collapsed across six electrode sites and nine consonant-vowel syllables that were recorded from 16 newborn infants whose language performance at age 3 years on the Stanford-Binet Verbal Reasoning subtest score was one standard deviation or more (range = 85–94) below the population mean (LOW group), the 47 infants who scored within one standard deviation (range = 95–116) of the population mean (AVERAGE group), and the 16 newborn infants who three years later scored one standard deviation or more (range = 117–130) above the population mean. The rectangle labeled factor 1 identifies the region of the ERP whose variability was reflected by factor 1 of the principal-components analysis. The region of variability characterized by factor 5 is demarcated by the rectangle that frames the later portion of the ERPS.

perform differently on a language-performance task. A similar effect was also reported by Molfese (1989) with a subset of the children involved in the current longitudinal study.

Interestingly, although it is generally believed that language perception is carried out by mechanisms within the left hemisphere (Lenneberg, 1967), variables reflecting recorded ERP activity across both hemispheres were used to successfully discriminate among these three groups of children in the current study. Prediction was not limited exclusively to the left-hemisphere electrode sites. These data could be used to argue that, at least in the early stages of postnatal life, the functioning of mechanisms within both hemispheres of the brain are important to later development.

From these findings it appears that electrophysiological measures obtained at birth involving the auditory event-related potential can be used successfully to discriminate between infants who three years later will display different levels of language skills. Obviously, these findings, if they continue to hold up as more children are followed into their later preschool and elementary-school years, may portend a radically new and highly accurate type of assessment tool. Finding such relationships between later cognitive skills and early neuroelectrical responses, though still tentative, could provide the basis for an early neuroelectrical screening test to identify children at birth or shortly after who may later have problems with language development. Such high predictive accuracy holds out the hope that very young infants who may be at risk for later cognitive or linguistic problems can be identified much earlier in development than is now thought possible. Consequently, intervention to address and perhaps remediate these disabilities could well start early in infancy, many years before our current assessment procedures now permit. If such potential problems can be identified and addressed early enough, it is possible that our success in remediating these problems will be greatly enhanced because we will be able to address these issues long before much of the cognitive and linguistics systems develop. We are continuing to follow our longitudinal sample through the middle-childhood years to determine whether the predictive accuracy—which currently appears very high—will continue to hold. We have also begun recruiting and testing yet another longitudinal sample to test whether the results from this current longitudinal study and that of Molfese and Molfese (1985) continue to hold up under further replication.

Acknowledgment. Support for this work was provided by the National Institutes of Health (R01 HD17860).

References

Blumstein, S.E., & Stevens, K.N. (1980). Perceptual invariance and onset spectra for stop consonants in different vowel environments. *Journal of the Acoustical Society of America, 66,* 1001–1017.

Bojean, C., Hill, R., & McLemore, S. (1967). *Sociological measurement: An inventory of scales and indices.* San Francisco: Chandler Publishing.

Brown, W.S., Marsh, J.T., & Smith, J.C. (1979). Principal component analysis of ERP differences related to the meaning of an ambiguous word. *Journal of Electroencephalography and Clinical Neurophysiology, 46,* 706–714.

Cattell, R.B. (1966). The scree test for the number of factors. *Multivariate Behavioral Research, 1,* 245.

Chapman, R.M., McCrary, J.W., Bragdon, H.R., & Chapman, J.A. (1979). Latent components of event-related potentials functionally related to information processing. In J.E. Desmedt (Ed.), *Progress in Clinical Neuropsychology, Vol. 6: Cognitive Components in Cerebral Event-Related Potentials and Selective Attention*. Basel: Karger.

Dixon, W.J. (Ed.) (1986). *BMDP Statistical Software 1986*. Berkeley: University of California Press.

Donchin, E., Tueting, P., Ritter, W., Kutas, M., & Heffley, E. (1975). On the independence of the CNV and the P300 components of the human averaged evoked potential. *Journal of Electroencephalography and Clinical Neurophysiology, 38,* 449–461.

Gelfer, M.P. (1987). An ERP study of stop-consonant discrimination. *Perception & Psychophysics, 42,* 318–327.

Jasper, H.H. (1958). The ten-twenty electrode system of the International Federation of Societies for Electroencephalography: Appendix to report of the committee on methods of clinical examination in electroencephalography. *Journal of Electroencephalography and Clinical Neurophysiology, 10,* 371–375.

Kaiser, H.F. (1958). The varimax criterion for analytic rotation in factor analysis. *Psychometrika, 23,* 187–200.

Lenneberg, E. (1967). *Biological Foundations of Language*. New York: Wiley.

McCarthy, D. (1972). *Manual for the McCarthy Scales of Children's Abilities*. New York: Psychological Corporation.

Molfese, D.L. (1978a). Electrophysiological correlates of categorical speech perception in adults. *Brain and Language, 5,* 25–35.

Molfese, D.L. (1978b). Left and right hemispheric involvement in speech perception: Electrophysiological correlates. *Perception & Psychophysics, 23,* 237–243.

Molfese, D.L. (1980). The phoneme and the engram: Electrophysiological evidence for the acoustic invariant in stop consonants. *Brain and Language, 9,* 372–376.

Molfese, D.L. (1984). Left hemisphere sensitivity to consonant sounds not displayed by the right hemisphere: Electrophysiological correlates. *Brain and Language, 22,* 109–127.

Molfese, D.L. (1988). *Evoked Potential Analysis and Collection System© (EPACS)*. U.S.A. Copyright.

Molfese, D.L. (1989). The use of auditory evoked responses recorded from newborn infants to predict later language skills. In N.W. Paul (Ed.), *Research in Infant Assessment*. White Plains, NY: Original Article Series, Vol. 25, No. 6, pp. 47–62.

Molfese, D.L. (1992). The use of auditory evoked responses recorded from newborn infants to predict language skills. In M.G. Tramontana & S.R. Hooper (Eds.), *Advances in Child Neuropsychology*, Vol. 1. New York: Springer-Verlag, pp. 1–23.

Molfese, D.L., & Molfese, V.J. (1979). Hemisphere and stimulus differences as reflected in the cortical responses of newborn infants to speech stimuli. *Developmental Psychology, 15,* 505–511.

Molfese, D.L., & Molfese, V.J. (1980). Cortical responses of preterm infants to phonetic and nonphonetic speech stimuli. *Developmental Psychology, 16,* 574–581.

Molfese, D.L., & Schmidt, A.L. (1983). An auditory evoked potential study of consonant perception. *Brain and Language, 18,* 57–70.

Molfese, D.L., & Molfese, V.J. (1985). Electrophysiological indices of auditory discrimination in newborn infants: The basis for predicting later language performance? *Infant Behavior and Development, 8,* 197–211.

Molfese, D.L., & Molfese, V.J. (1993). *Brain Responses at Birth Predict Language Skills at Three Years-of-Age. A Longitudinal Study.* Chicago: Midwestern Psychological Association.

Oldfield, R.L. (1971). The assessment of handedness: The Edinburgh Inventory. *Neuropsychologia, 9,* 97–113.

Rockstroh, B., Elbert, T., Birbaumer, N., & Lutzenberger, W. (1982). *Slow brain potentials and behavior.* Baltimore: Urban & Schwarzenberg.

Ruchkin, D., Sutton, S., Munson, R., Silver, K., & Macar, F. (1981). P300 and feedback provided by absence of the stimulus. *Psychophysiology, 18,* 271–282.

Segalowitz, S.J., & Cohen, H. (1989). Right hemisphere EEG sensitivity to speech. *Brain and Language, 37,* 220–231.

Thorndike, R.L., Hagen, E.P., & Sattler, J.M. (1986). *Stanford-Binet Intelligence Scale.* 4th Ed. Chicago: Riverside Publishing.

CHAPTER 2

Lead and Neuropsychological Function in Children: Progress and Problems in Establishing Brain–Behavior Relationships

DAVID BELLINGER

Lead is a ubiquitous environmental pollutant whose contribution to the pathogenesis of numerous human diseases has long been recognized, albeit not completely understood (NRC, 1993). Surprisingly, knowledge about lead's devastating influence on the developing central nervous system dates only from the end of the nineteenth century (Gibson, Love, Hardine, Bancroft, & Turner, 1892). In their case series, a benchmark investigation in this literature, Byers and Lord (1943) demonstrated that lead poisoning need not progress to frank encephalopathy (i.e., cerebral edema and hemorrhage) for children to experience severe intellectual and behavioral sequelae. This discovery spawned worry over "low-level" or subclinical lead exposures, those within the range of exposures that may be incurred by residence in a modern industrial setting but not high enough to produce classic symptoms of lead poisoning. The hypothesis that such exposures impair children's mental function has been a topic of spirited, often acrimonious debate since the 1970s.

The quantity of data on sources and pathways of human lead exposure, population blood lead levels, and dose-response relationships for a spectrum of health effects is unparalleled among environmental toxicants. The results of risk-assessment analyses can thus be stated with greater certainty than can analyses of other toxicants, requiring fewer extrapolations from animal models to human beings or from high-dose to low-dose scenarios. Examining the data on lead's effects on neurobehavioral development may identify principles and lessons germane to investigating other neurotoxic pollutants, such as polychlorinated biphenyls (Tilson, Jacobson, & Rogan, 1990), methylmercury (Burbacher, Rodier, & Weiss, 1990), and pesticides (Davies, 1990).

The thesis to be developed is that available data, collected primarily with a public-health goal, are sufficient for major revisions in guidelines for lead screening and treatment policy but leave significant lacunae in our understanding of lead's effect on children's nervous systems. With the overriding goal of providing an answer to the practical question of what levels produce detectable changes in children's behavior, investigators have generally chosen to employ behavioral endpoints that are familiar, easily communicated, and psychometrically sound, and to recruit study cohorts with lead levels at or below current screening targets. These circumstances generally will not generate data explicating the neuropsychological underpinnings of lead's effect on intellectual and academic function, and it is unreasonable to criticize them for failing to do so.

In this chapter we describe the findings of a prospective study of lead exposure and child development conducted by our group in Boston and use them as a springboard for discussing major gaps in our understanding of lead neurotoxicity. No attempt is made to survey the extensive literature, because several recent comprehensive reviews are available (Bellinger & Dietrich, in press; Needleman & Bellinger, 1991; U.S. EPA, 1990). To set the context, however, we review briefly the evidence that such an association exists at all, after adjustment for potential confounding bias. When a health endpoint that is the final common pathway for many sociocultural as well as chemical exposures can be studied only by means of observational designs, distinguishing the contribution of the factor of interest from those of correlated risk factors is fraught with ambiguity. The intensity of the resulting debate is heightened when policy decisions with substantial economic implications must be based on evidence that is necessarily incomplete. Dozens of studies of lead and children's IQ have been conducted and overall trends in the findings have been described with various meta-analytic methods. Needleman and Gatsonis (1990) concluded that the mean partial (i.e., adjusted) correlation between blood lead level and IQ in the major cross-sectional studies was −0.15 (95% confidence interval (CI): −0.10, −0.20). The mean partial correlation between tooth lead level and IQ was −0.08 (95% CI: −0.03, −0.13). Schwartz (in press) evaluated the consistency in study findings from the standpoint of adjusted regression coefficients (i.e., the change in IQ per unit of increase in lead-exposure index). Combining the findings of cross-sectional and prospective studies, he estimated the common effect size (ES) to be a decline of 2.6 IQ points (SE = 0.4) for an increase in blood lead concentration from 10 to 20 micrograms per deciliter (μg/dL). Surprisingly similar estimates were derived for prospective (2.3 points) and cross-sectional studies (2.7 points). In a meta-analysis included in the most recent revision of the World Health Organization's *Environmental Health Criteria for Inorganic Lead* (WHO, in press), the ES based on prospective studies for the relationship between mean postnatal blood lead level and IQ at school age was −2.0 points (95% CI: −0.3, −3.6; $p = 0.01$) for an increase from 10 to 20 μg/dL. The effect size estimated from cross-sectional studies was similar (−2.1 points, 95% CI: −1.2, −3.1; $p < 0.001$). The conclusion of the WHO Task Group was that, "The size of the apparent IQ effect (at age 4 and above) is a deficit between 0 and 5 points (on a scale with a standard deviation of 15) for each 10 μg/dL increment in blood lead level, with a likely apparent effect size of between 1 and 3 points. Below the range of 10 to 15 µg/dL, the effect of confounding variables and limits in the precision of analytical and psychometric measurements increases the uncertainty attached to any estimate of effect."

In aggregate, then, available data strongly support a significant but modest inverse association between low-level lead and IQ. Some, but not all observers have concluded that the relationship is likely to be causal (Schwartz, in press; Thacker, Hoffman, Smith, Steinberg, & Zack, 1992). The former Secretary of the U.S. Department of Health and Human Services, Louis Sullivan, recently identified lead poisoning as the major environmental health problem of U.S. children (Sullivan, 1991) and announced another in a series of downward revisions made over the past 25 years in the blood lead level considered worth worrying about (Centers for Disease Control, 1991). Late in the 1960s, a blood lead level of 60 µg/dL was considered the upper limit of normal for children. By 1985, it had been redefined as 25 µg/dL. At present, a blood lead level greater than 10 µg/dL is considered "lead poisoning," and various nutritional, environmental, and medical interventions are recommended at levels of 15 and 20 µg/dL. The CDC states, however, that no blood lead level may be safe—i.e., no threshold level below which adverse health effects do not occur. Although population blood lead levels have dropped precipitously in the United States in the last two decades (Annest, Pirkle, Makuc, Neese, Bayse, & Kovar, 1983), the average body burden remains several orders of magnitude higher than the human "natural background" level, calculated from geochemical evidence (Flegal & Smith, 1992). Thus, today's "average" does not necessarily mean "physiologically normal." The mean blood lead level among U.S. children is currently estimated to be 4 to 6 µg/dL.

The Boston Prospective Study

Recognizing limitations on the inferences that can be drawn from retrospective or cross-sectional studies (Bellinger & Stiles, 1993), several groups began prospective studies around 1980, serially measuring both lead burden and postnatal neurobehavioral development. The sites of these studies are Boston, Cincinnati (Dietrich, Krafft, Bornschein, Hammond, Berger, Succop, & Bier, 1987; Dietrich, Succop, Bornschein, Krafft, Berger, Hammond, & Buncher, 1990; Dietrich, Succop, Berger, Hammond, & Bornschein, 1991; Dietrich, Succop, Berger, & Keith, 1992; Dietrich, Berger, & Succop, 1993a; Dietrich, Berger, Succop, & Hammond, 1993b), Port Pirie, South Australia (Baghurst, McMichael, Wigg, Vimpani, Robertson, Roberts, & Tong, 1992; McMichael, Baghurst, Wigg, Vimpani, Robertson, & Roberts, 1988; Wigg, Vimpani, McMichael, Baghurst, Robertson, & Roberts, 1988), Cleveland (Ernhart, Morrow-

Tlucak, Marler, & Wolf, 1987; Ernhart, Morrow-Tlucak, Wolf, Super, & Drotar, 1989), Sydney (Cooney, Bell, McBride, & Carter 1989a, 1989b), Kosovo (Serbia) (Wasserman, Graziano, Factor-Litvak, Popovac, Morina, Musabegovic, Vrenezi, Capuni-Paracka, Lekic, Preteni-Redjepi, Hadzialjevic, Slavkovich, Kline, Shrout, & Stein, 1992), and Mexico City (Rothenberg, Lourdes, Cansino-Ortiz, Perroni-Hernandez, de la Torre, Neri-Mendez, Ortega, Hidalgo-Loperena, & Svensgaard, 1989).

To assemble a study cohort in Boston, our group collected umbilical-cord blood samples from nearly 12,000 babies (approximately 97% of the deliveries) born between April 1979 and March 1980 at the Boston Lying-In Division of the Boston Hospital for Women (now Brigham and Women's Hospital) (Rabinowitz & Needleman, 1982). Reasoning that oversampling children with cord blood lead levels in the extremes of the distribution would provide the greatest statistical power to detect any effect prenatal lead exposure might have on development, we recruited 3 groups of children for study: 85 with cord blood lead levels below the 10th percentile for this delivery population ($<3\,\mu g/dL$), 88 with levels close to the mean ($6\,\mu g/dL$), and 76 with levels greater than the 90th percentile ($\geq 10\,\mu g/dL$ but less than $25\,\mu g/dL$). The sampling frames for other studies differed, recruiting consecutive registrants for prenatal care or women with specific characteristics of interest (e.g., history of alcohol abuse). In many of these cohorts, the distribution of prenatal lead exposures more closely reflects the distribution in the source population, with relatively few individuals having extremely high or extremely low exposures. This balance reflects a trade-off between generalizability and statistical power. Although other cohorts may better assess population-attributable risk, the reduced number of participants with extreme exposures provides relatively lower power to detect subtle developmental influence of mildly elevated prenatal exposures.

We excluded from our cohort children with medical conditions known to be associated with increased risk of developmental handicap (e.g., gestational age <34 weeks, Down Syndrome) (see Bellinger, Needleman, Leviton, Waternaux, Rabinowitz, & Nichols, 1984 for additional information on recruitment). In general, the cohort consisted of healthy neonates from middle- and upper-middle-class backgrounds. The decision to sample children at low risk of developmental problems was based on the epidemiologic principle that a small effect (the "signal") is easier to detect when the prevalence of competing risks (the "noise") for the outcome of interest is low, producing a high signal-to-noise ratio (Rothman & Poole, 1988). Increased lead exposure generally occurs along with many other poverty-related developmental risks (Mahaffey, Annest, Roberts, & Murphy, 1982). Deciding how to apportion outcome variance among correlated risk factors is a formidable task, creating conditions ripe for committing both Type I and Type II errors (Bellinger & Stiles, 1993). In a series of simulation analyses, we found that the likelihood of "detecting" an association of given magnitude can vary substantially depending on the correlations among lead burden, IQ, and a potential confounder (Bellinger, Leviton, & Waternaux, 1989). Therefore, just as epidemiologists interested in contributions by airborne pollutants to lung cancer may restrict the study population to nonsmokers (Mills, Abbey, Beeson, & Peterson, 1991), we selected as our target population children presumed to be functioning near their maximum potential because other significant developmental risk factors were relatively absent (Bellinger, Leviton, Rabinowitz, Needleman, & Waternaux, 1986).

Estimates of postnatal lead exposure were provided by measuring the concentration of lead in blood obtained by finger stick at ages 6, 12, 18, and 24 months, and by venipuncture at ages 57 months and 10 years. The mean concentration never exceeded 8 μg/dL, although at each sampling age except for 10 years, a few children had blood lead levels in excess of 20 μg/dL. The children's blood lead profiles did not reflect the phenomenon of "blood lead tracking" (i.e., high intraindividual stability in blood lead level) to the extent seen in many high-risk cohorts (Baghurst et al., 1992; Dietrich et al., 1993b). This relative lack of confounding of exposures during different developmental epochs afforded us a better opportunity to identify periods of increased vulnerability than is provided when blood lead is highly stable.

Children's general developmental and intellectual status was assessed at ages 6, 12, 18, and 24 months using the Bayley Scales of Infant Development, at age 57 months using McCarthy Scales of Children's Abilities, and at 10 years using the Wechsler Intelligence Scale for Children-Revised (WISC-R). Additional assessments were included at each age. The children consistently performed at a high level. Both Mental Developmental Index (MDI) scores at 24 months and General Cognitive Index (GCI) scores at 57 months averaged approximately 115. The mean WISC-R Full-Scale IQ at 10 years was 119.

Results of Assessments During Infancy

Children with "high" cord blood lead levels (i.e., ≥10 μg/dL) achieved covariate-adjusted MDI scores that were 4 to 8 points lower than those of children with "low" cord blood lead levels at ages 6, 12, 18, and 24 months (Bellinger et al., 1984; Bellinger, Leviton, Needleman, Waternaux, & Rabinowitz, 1986; Bellinger, Leviton, Waternaux, Needleman, & Rabinowitz, 1987) (Figure 2.1). In regression analyses, adjustments were made for maternal age, race, maternal IQ, maternal education, smoking history, alcohol consumption during pregnancy, family social class, Home Observation for Measurement of the Environment (HOME) score, gender, birthweight, gestational age, and birth order. The MDI scores were not associated with blood lead levels measured postnatally, leading us to infer that the persistent performance differences

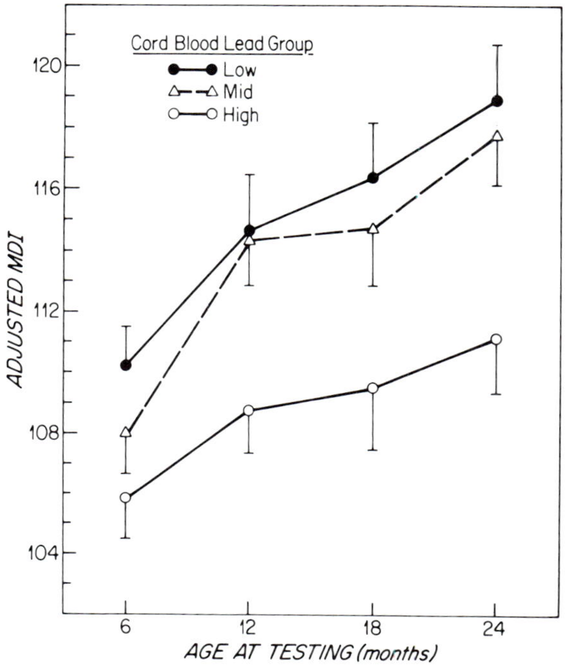

Fig. 2.1. Adjusted mean Mental Development Index scores at 4 postnatal ages of children classified by umbilical cord blood-lead level (low: <3 μg/dL; mid: 6 to 7 μg/dL; high: ≥10 μg/dL). Error bars represent one standard error. (Reprinted by permission of the *New England Journal of Medicine* (vol. 316, page 1041, 1987).)

were attributable to differing levels of in utero exposure. Additional analyses, varying aspects of the statistical adjustment, suggested that this finding was robust to differences in strategy for selecting potential confounders for which to adjust (viz., empirical or subject-matter based), differences in methods of refining the multivariate model (viz., backward stepwise, optimal, or all-subsets regression), and differences in ways of parameterizing prenatal lead exposure (viz., continuously distributed variable, natural log transform, ordered or unordered dummy variables) (Bellinger, Leviton, Waternaux, & Allred, 1985; Bellinger, Leviton, Waternaux, Needleman, & Rabinowitz, 1989).

In animal studies of behavioral toxicants, clear individual differences in the magnitude of "response" to the same dose are frequently reported (e.g., Rice, 1992a). Because environmental regulations are often formulated to provide adequate protection to the most vulnerable subgroups in a population, it is important to determine whether lead is more detrimental to some infants than others and, if so, to identify biologic or environmental correlates of response variability. To date, the primary

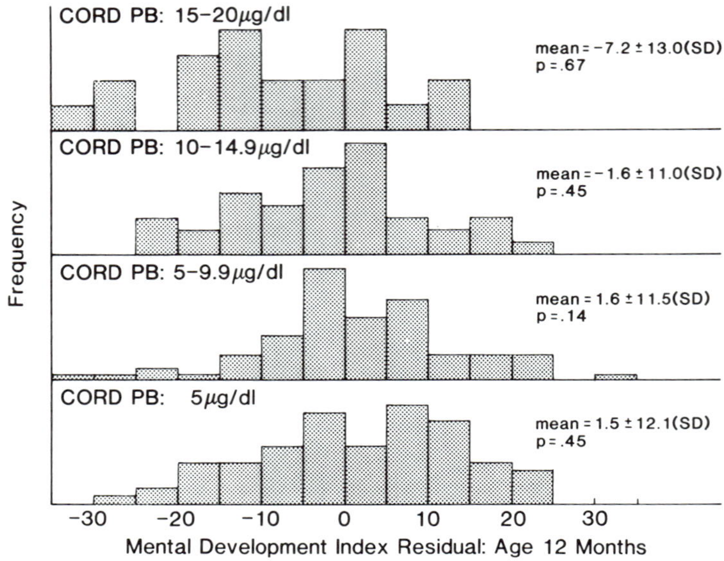

Fig. 2.2. Histograms of Mental Development Index residual scores at age 12 months of children classified by umbilical-cord blood-lead level. *P*-value to the right of each distribution refers to null hypothesis that the distribution of residual scores is normal. (Reprinted by permission of the March of Dimes Foundation.)

goal in lead research has been to describe overall population risks rather than to ascertain characteristics that determine an individual child's risk. In attempting to address the first issue, we reasoned that if the lower mean score of the "high" cord blood lead group was due to the inordinate influence of a small subset of especially sensitive children, the distribution of "developmental responses" within this group should be bimodal. In contrast, a normal distribution of responses would suggest that this group's lower mean score reflected a tendency for the performance of most children to be affected, but to an extent that varied randomly. To quantify "response" to a given lead burden, we calculated a predicted MDI score for each child at age 12 months based on medical and sociodemographic factors that generally correlate with infant development. Residual scores were derived by subtracting a child's predicted score from the MDI score he or she achieved, and the distributions of residual scores plotted for children in 4 cord blood lead strata, 0–4.9, 5.0–9.9, 10.0–14.9, and ≥15 μg/dL (Figure 2.2). Within each stratum, the distribution of residual scores did not deviate significantly from normality, failing to support the hypothesis that the lower mean performance of children with "high" cord blood lead reflects heterogeneity in responses by the children within this group. Rather, the data suggest that once adjustments are made for potential confounders, individual differences in putative influence of lead

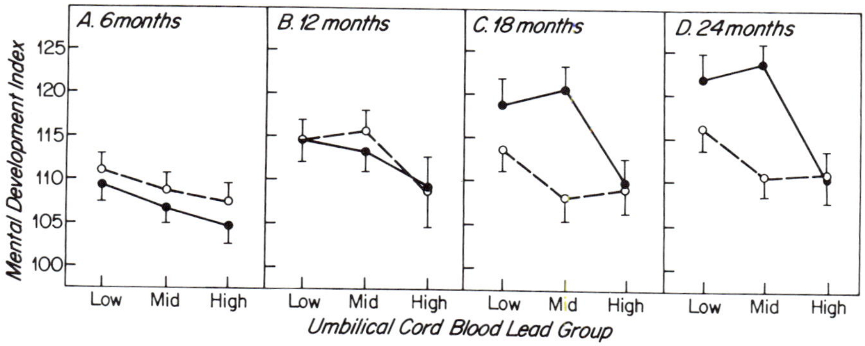

Fig. 2.3. Adjusted Mental Development Index scores at 4 postnatal ages of children classified by umbilical-cord blood-lead (low, mid, high) and social class (median split). Open circles represent children from families below the median social class. Closed circles represent children from families above the median social class. Error bars represent one standard error. (Reprinted from *Neurotoxicology and Teratology*, Vol. 10, Bellinger et al., Low-level lead exposure, social class, and infant development, pp. 497–503, Copyright 1988, with kind permission from Pergamon Press Ltd, Headington Hill Hall, Oxford OX3 OBW, UK.)

are randomly distributed about a value that is a meaningful descriptor of the "average" response to a given lead dose (Bellinger & Needleman, 1992).

The second issue we sought to address was the extent to which variation in "response" magnitude was associated with child characteristics. Numerous studies document how social factors influence developmental prognosis following early biologic insult (Aylward, 1992), and we observed a similar phenomenon in our data (Bellinger, Leviton, Waternaux, Needleman, & Rabinowitz, 1988). The association between MDI scores and cord blood lead category was examined separately by social-class strata (below median vs. above median). At age 6 and 12 months, the association was similar across groups (Figures 2.3A,B), as expected because social class tends not to predict development until the second year of life (Golden & Birns, 1983). At age 18 and 24 months, however, a significant cord blood lead × social class interaction was found (Figures 2.3C,D). The scores of children below the median social class declined at "medium" blood lead levels, suggesting increased vulnerability among these children compared to those above the median social class. No social-class differences were apparent among children with cord blood lead levels greater than 10 μg/dL, however, suggesting that lead's influence was sufficient to override whatever it is about membership in the upper half of the social-class distribution that enables children to perform better on developmental tests than their less privileged peers. Several studies suggest that lead effects may be more prominent among lower-class children (Dietrich, Krafft, Bornschein, Hammond, Berger, Succop, & Bier, 1987, 1991; Lansdown, Yule, Urbanowicz, & Hunter, 1986; Harvey, Hamlin, Kumar, & Delves, 1984; Winneke & Kramer, 1984), although others do not (Pocock, Ashby, & Smith, 1987). As-yet unidentified methodological factors may also be responsible (e.g., cohort characteristics such as general level and dispersion of social-class scores, or characteristics of exposure profiles).

Results of Assessments at Preschool Age

Contrary to our findings during infancy, an association between prenatal lead exposure and cognitive performance was not evident at age 57 months when the McCarthy Scales of Children's Abilities were administered ($N = 169$). The adjusted General Cognitive Index (GCI) scores of children with "high" ($\geq 10\,\mu g/dL$) cord blood lead levels (116.2, SE = 1.8) were indistinguishable from the scores of children with either "low" (117.6, SE = 1.8) or "medium" levels (114.6, SE = 1.7) (Bellinger, Sloman, Leviton, Rabinowitz, Needleman, & Waternaux, 1991). Thus, in a cohort with substantial socioeconomic advantages, any influence of elevated prenatal exposure may be transient. The other prospective studies also failed to find a significant association between prenatal exposure and cognitive function in the preschool period or beyond.

Additional analyses suggested that the developmental prognosis associated with high prenatal exposure may vary depending on factors such as level of postnatal lead exposure and sociodemographic indicators (Bellinger, Leviton, & Sloman, 1990). Among the children with cord blood lead levels $\geq 10\,\mu g/dL$, change in performance between 24 and 57 months (the difference between MDI at 24 months and GCI at 57 months) was dose-related to blood lead level measured at 57 months (Figure 2.4). Consider two children who had high cord blood lead levels and who achieved the same MDI score at age 24 months. If one child had a low ($\leq 3\,\mu g/dL$) blood lead level at 57 months and the other had a high ($\geq 10\,\mu g/dL$) level, our model predicted that the GCI score of the child with the higher blood lead level would be 9.1 points lower than the score of the child with the lower blood lead level. The dependence of performance change on concurrent lead level was much less striking among children with either low or medium cord blood lead levels. "Recovery from" or "compensation for" the adverse developmental influence of high prenatal lead exposure also was greater among children with more optimal sociodemographic characteristics such as higher social-class standing, higher maternal IQ, higher HOME scores, and female gender.

Although a main-effect association between prenatal exposure and preschool performance was not evident at 57 months, adjusted GCI scores were inversely related to postnatal blood lead levels. Only for the

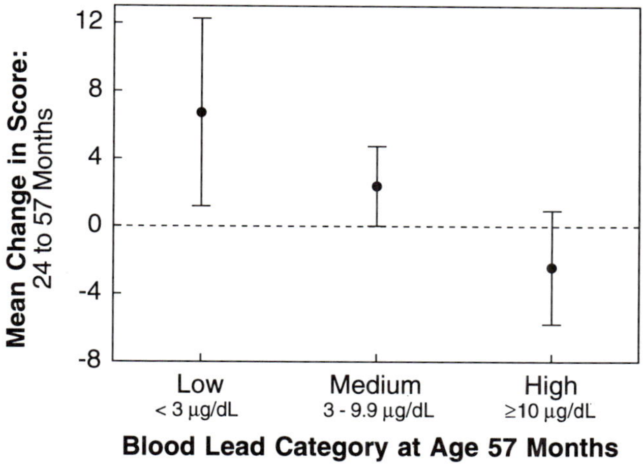

Fig. 2.4. Mean change in performance between 57 and 24 months among children who had high umbilical-cord blood-lead levels (≥10 µg/dL), stratified by blood lead level at age 57 months. "Change in performance" is defined as adjusted General Cognitive Index score at 57 months minus adjusted Mental Development Index score at 24 months. Error bars represent one standard error. (Reproduced by permission of *Pediatrics* (vol. 87, p. 225, Copyright 1991) (modified).)

level measured at age 2 years, however, was the association statistically significant (Figure 2.5). In regression analyses, adjustment was made for social class, maternal IQ, maternal marital status, preschool attendance, HOME score, amount of out-of-home care, changes in family residence, use of medication, number of adults in household, gender, race, birthweight, and birth order. Children with low blood lead levels at age 2 years (<3 µg/dL) had GCI scores that were on average 6.4 points higher than those of children with "high" (≥10 µg/dL) blood lead levels at 2 years. This association was due largely to the lower scores of more highly exposed children on the Perceptual-Performance subscale of the McCarthy Scales. Blood lead level at 57 months also was inversely and significantly associated with scores on this subscale. Overall, the mean 2-year blood lead level of the children who participated at 57 months was quite modest, 6.8 µg/dL (SD = 6.3, 90th percentile = 13.7).

Results of Assessments at School Age

A battery of standardized psychometric and neuropsychologic tests was administered to 148 of the children remaining in the cohort at age 10 years. To structure our interpretation of the many test results anticipated and to reduce the risk of Type I error, we designated scores on the Wechsler Intelligence Scale for Children-Revised (WISC-R) and the

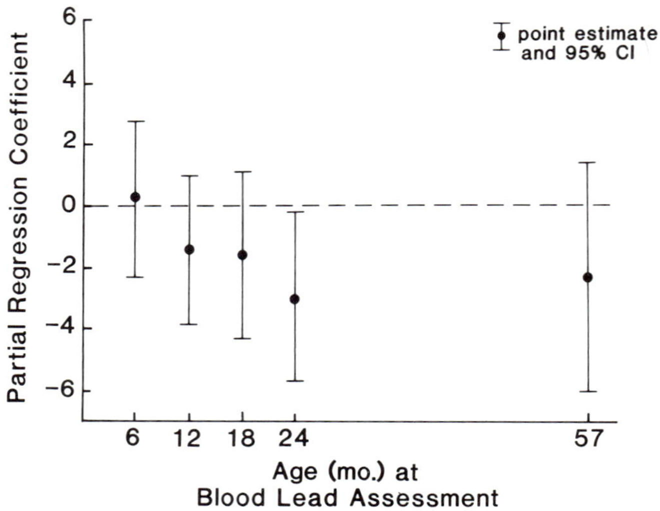

Fig. 2.5. Adjusted regression coefficients (point estimates) for blood-lead levels at 5 postnatal ages and General Cognitive Index score at 57 months. Error bars represent the 95% confidence intervals for the point estimates. (Reprinted by permission of *Neurotoxicology* (vol. 14, p. 155, 1993).)

Kaufman-Test of Educational Achievement (K-TEA) as the primary endpoints. The other tests administered were viewed as secondary, to help formulate hypotheses about the neuropsychological underpinnings of any lead-associated differences seen in WISC-R and K-TEA scores. These tests included the Rey-Osterreith Complex Figure (ROCF), the California Verbal Learning Test for Children (CVLT-C), the Developmental Test of Visual-Motor Integration, finger tapping, story memory, and the Grooved Pegboard.

The results of the 10-year assessments were startling. Many scores on the primary outcome measures at age 10 years, like scores on the McCarthy Scales at age 57 months, were inversely related to blood lead level measured at age 2 years (Figure 2.6) (Bellinger, Stiles, & Needleman, 1992). An increase of 10 μg/dL in blood lead level at age 2 was associated with a decrement of 5.8 points in WISC-R full-scale IQ (95% CI: 1.7 to 9.9, $p = 0.007$), and a deficit of 8.9 points in K-TEA Battery Composite (95% CI: 4.2 to 13.6, $p = 0.0003$). These estimates were adjusted for HOME scores at 57 months and 10 years (selected scales), child stress, maternal age, race, maternal IQ, socioeconomic status, gender, birth order, maternal marital status, and number of changes in family residence. The association was stronger for Verbal IQ than for Performance IQ, and stronger for spelling and mathematics achievement than for reading achievement.

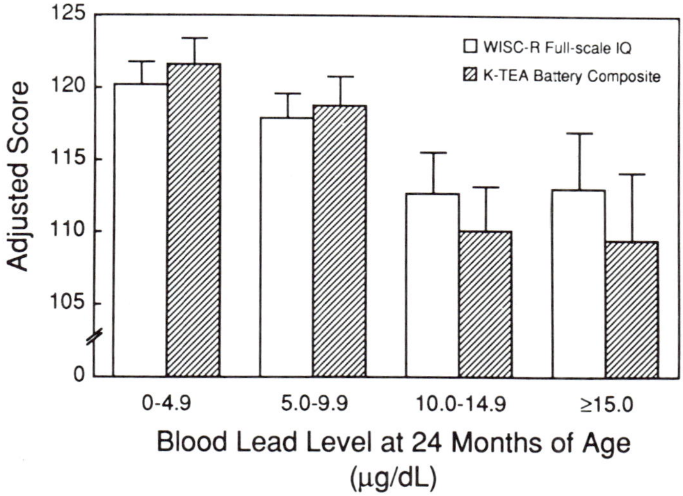

Fig. 2.6. Adjusted mean Full-Scale WISC-R IQ and Battery Composite scores on the Kaufman-Test of Educational Achievement of children stratified by blood-lead level at 2 years of age. Error bars represent one standard error. (Reproduced by permission of *Pediatrics* (vol. 90, p. 858, Copyright 1992).)

Because of the surprising magnitude of these putative lead effects and their apparent persistence over several years, various additional analyses were carried out to evaluate methodological and substantive factors that might have produced spurious associations. Inspecting partial regression residual plots and considering nonlinear models using nonparametric smoothing methods provided no indication of a threshold for the association (Schwartz, 1994). Various sensitivity analyses indicated that the results were not substantially affected by deleting cases identified as influential because of their residuals, their effect on regression coefficients, or their effect on fitted values.

Because 2-year blood lead level was significantly associated with GCI at 57 months, which in turn was correlated with IQ at 10 years, we included GCI score in the regression model. The association between IQ at 10 years and 2-year blood lead level remained significant. Several explanations for this finding are possible. The GCI scores at 57 months may not reflect the complete spectrum of lead's adverse influence on children's intellectual function, either because of restrictions in coverage of primary neuropsychological domains or because of lower test sensitivity. Alternatively, "new" lead effects may continue to be expressed between 57 months and 10 years as the toxicologic effect continues. Similar increases over time in the magnitude of apparent effects were recorded by Achenbach, Howell, Aoki, and Rauh (1993) in a randomized trial of a short-term intervention designed to facilitate the interaction between low-birthweight infants and their mothers, and by Aylward (1993) in studying indicators of perinatal asphyxia (e.g., arterial pH, $PACO_2$) and later development.

To evaluate the issue of age-dependent vulnerability, we explored different ways of integrating the serial blood lead levels. The regression coefficient associated with the average of the 24- and 57-month blood lead levels was substantially greater than the coefficient associated with 2-year blood lead alone (−0.82 vs. −0.58), although it was estimated with less precision (standard error of 0.28 vs. 0.21). In most cohorts, the high intraindividual blood lead stability ("blood lead tracking") and the confounding of age and peak blood lead level (around age 2 years) impede efforts to identify periods of heightened sensitivity to lead. Although peak blood lead level occurred at an age other than 2 years for many children in our cohort, blood lead level measured at 2 years was nevertheless more strongly related to IQ at 10 years than was the maximum level measured. This finding implicates the period around age 2 years as a time when the nervous system may be especially vulnerable to disruption by lead.

Efforts to identify specific neuropsychological processes that underlie the global deficits observed in IQ and educational achievement were disappointing (Stiles & Bellinger, 1993). Several WISC-R subtest scores were inversely associated with 2-year blood lead level (Table 2.1), particularly those contributing to verbal IQ. Verbal IQ–Performance IQ discrepancies of 12 or more points were significantly less frequent among children with 2-year lead levels greater than 10 μg/dL. Similarly, the amount of subtest scatter (i.e., the number of subtest scores differing from the subtest mean score by 3 or more standard units) was unrelated

Table 2.1. WISC-R scores: Adjusted regression coefficients associated with blood lead at age 2 years.

Score	Coefficient[a]	Standard error	*P*-value
Information	−0.07	0.05	0.13
Similarities	−0.13	0.05	0.011
Arithmetic	−0.12	0.04	0.010
Vocabulary	−0.08	0.04	0.090
Comprehension	−0.10	0.04	0.018
Digit Span	−0.09	0.05	0.056
Picture Completion	−0.09	0.04	0.030
Picture Arrangement	0.02	0.05	0.63
Block Design	−0.11	0.06	0.043
Object Assembly	−0.05	0.05	0.29
Coding	−0.05	0.05	0.35
Mazes	−0.04	0.05	0.46

[a] Coefficient represents the estimated change in score associated with each 1 μg/dL increase in blood-lead level at age 2 years.

Source: Adapted from Stiles and Bellinger (1993).

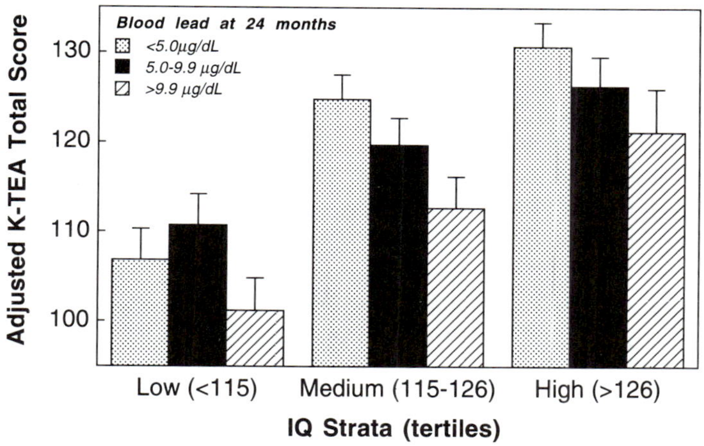

Fig. 2.7. Adjusted Battery Composite scores on the Kaufman-Test of Educational Achievement for children stratified by blood-lead level at 2 years of age and by Full-Scale WISC-R IQ at 10 years of age. Error bars represent one standard error.

to 2-year blood lead. In multivariate regression analyses, 2-year blood lead level was associated with scores on the Freedom from Distractibility Factor (Arithmetic, Digit Span, Coding), although not with Verbal Comprehension or Perceptual Organization factor scores. Although a few significant associations were found between 2-year blood lead and various dependent variables from the neuropsychological tests (e.g., CVLT-C perseveration score, story recall, ROCF copy organization score, number of pegs dropped with nonpreferred hand on Grooved Pegboard), they did not describe a coherent pattern, nor did the number of associations exceed that expected by chance. The IQ scores alone clearly did not capture the entirety of lead's apparent influence, however, because the association between 2-year blood lead and K-TEA Battery Composite remained significant when IQ was controlled statistically. Even among children with IQs nearly 2 standard deviations above the expected population mean, 2-year blood lead level was clearly associated with lower battery composite scores (Figure 2.7).

Characterizing the Neuropsychological Target(s) of Lead

Our inability to discern a behavioral or neuropsychological "signature" for lead is not unique. Although most studies provide evidence of an association between increased lead exposure and poorer performance in some neuropsychological domain, the lack of consistency across studies in the specific domains and in the pattern of performance decrements is more striking than any similarities.

It is even difficult to conclude whether the influence of higher exposures is generally greater in the verbal or nonverbal domain. In some studies lead is more strongly associated with verbal IQ (or a surrogate score) than with performance IQ (Baghurst, McMichael, Wigg, Vimpani, Robertson, Roberts, & Tong, 1992; Bellinger, Stiles, & Needleman, 1992; Bergomi, Borella, Fantuzzi, Vivoli, Sturloni, Cavazzuti, Tampieri, & Tartoni, 1989; Ernhart, Landa, & Schell, 1981; Hansen, Trillingsgaard, Beese, Lyngbye, & Grandjean, 1989; Needleman, Gunnoe, Leviton, Reed, Peresie, Maher, & Barrett, 1979; Yule, Lansdown, Millar, & Urbanowicz, 1981), but in other studies the pattern is reversed (Dietrich, Berger, Succop, & Hammond, 1993b; Marecek, Shapiro, Burke, Katz, & Hediger, 1983; Shapiro & Marecek, 1984). In yet other studies, lead is significantly associated with both (Hatzakis, Kokkevi, Maravelias, Katsouyanni, Salaminios, Kalandidi, Koutselinis, Stefanis, & Trichopoulos, 1989) or with neither (Fergusson, Fergusson, Horwood, & Kinzett, 1988; Lansdown, Yule, Urbanowicz, & Hunter, 1986; Silva, Hughes, Williams, & Faed, 1988; Smith, Delves, Lansdown, Clayton, & Graham, 1983; Winneke, Kramer, Brockhaus, Ewers, Kujanek, Lechner, & Janke, 1983). Several studies have found significant lead-associated decrements on tests of visual-spatial and visual-motor integration (Bellinger, Sloman, Leviton, Rabinowitz, Needleman, & Waternaux, 1991; Dietrich, Berger, & Succop, 1993a; Hansen, Trillingsgaard, Beese, Lyngbye, & Grandjean, 1989; McMichael, Baghurst, Wigg, Vimpani, Robertson, & Roberts, 1988; Winneke, Brockhaus, Ewers, Kramer, & Neuf, 1990). Perhaps the most consistent finding is poorer performance on simple or choice reaction-time tasks by children with greater lead burdens (Hatzakis, Kokkevi, Maravelias, Katsouyanni, Salaminios, Kalandi, Koutselinis, Stefanis, & Trichopoulos, 1989; Hunter, Urbanowicz, Yule, & Lansdown, 1985; Needleman, Gunnoe, Leviton, Reed, Peresie, Maher, & Barret, 1979; Needleman, Schell, Bellinger, Leviton, & Allred, 1990; Raab, Thomson, Boyd, Fulton, & Laxen, 1990; Winneke, Kramer, Brockhaus, Ewers, Kujanek, Lechner, & Janke, 1983; Winneke, Brockhaus, Collet, & Kramer, 1989).

The absence of a "signature" syndrome of neuropsychological deficit has troubled many observers, leading them to question if the associations seen on global indices reflect a causal role for lead. In drawing inferences from data about possible brain–behavior relationships underlying low-level lead toxicity, however, it is critical to consider (1) the toxicokinetics of lead, (2) lead-environment interactions, and (3) the developmental effects of lead on nervous-system morphology and physiology.

Toxicokinetics

It seems likely that attempts to identify the neuropsychologic functions most vulnerable to lead will not succeed unless important parameters of children's exposures are characterized more accurately and thoroughly

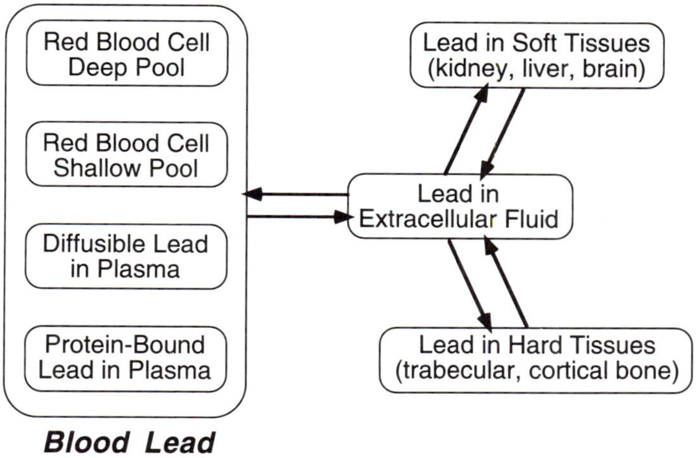

Fig. 2.8. Schematic representation of a compartmental model of body lead burden. (Adapted from Figure 10-4 in U.S. EPA (1986a), based on Marcus (1985).)

than has been achieved in studies to date. Lead is a multimedia pollutant and exposure occurs throughout an individual's lifetime, although the relative importance of sources changes. Internal dose at any one time will vary with intrinsic factors such as age, past exposures, and genetics, and with extrinsic factors such as location and age of residence, occupation, and patterns of activity. This variability can create substantial difficulties in classifying the individual's exposure, a problem that is exacerbated by the complexities in lead metabolism (absorption, distribution, and excretion). The concentration of lead in blood is the most frequently used index of body burden, and yet under most exposure scenarios a blood lead level mostly reflects recent exposure. The residence time of lead in blood is relatively short (a half-life of approximately a month). Most of the lead in blood (~95%) is bound to red cells, yet it is the remaining 5%, found in plasma, which is thought to be the biologically active fraction. From blood, lead moves into soft and hard tissues as shown in Figure 2.8, a schematic representation of the major body compartments or pools of lead in the body. Lead in the various pools is in dynamic equilibrium and can be redistributed depending on changes in external exposure or on the occurrence of various pathologic states (e.g., demineralization of bone because of traumatic injury, infection, or immobilization) and physiologic changes (e.g., pregnancy, menopause, and age- or growth-related bone remodeling processes) (Silbergeld, 1991).

The complexity of lead pharmacokinetics has several implications. A blood lead level taken at one time, frequently the sole measure of body burden available in a cross-sectional study, may be misleading. A low current level could mask substantial past exposures, and thus the presence of large amounts of potentially mobilizable lead in other pools, especially bone. Misclassification of children's exposure will generally bias assessments of the association between lead and neuropsychological performance toward the null hypothesis. At best, it will distort estimates of dose-response relationships. For this and other reasons, great efforts have recently been made to develop X-ray fluorescence-based methods for in vivo (noninvasive) measurement of lead in bone as an index of cumulative exposure (Nordberg, Mahaffey, & Fowler, 1991). Another form of exposure misclassification may result because lead concentration in peripheral blood may not always correlate highly with the concentration at critical organ sites, such as the brain. The relationship between blood lead and brain lead levels under different exposure scenarios is not well understood, but in animal models brain lead does not decrease as rapidly as blood lead following chelation or cessation of exposure (Goldstein, Asbury, & Diamond, 1974).

There are other dangers to ignoring important pharmacokinetic factors. In analyzing data from a cross-sectional study, all children with a specified blood lead level are assumed to be equally exposed, even though details of their past exposures may bear little similarity. One child may have had a few "spikes" of acute high-lead exposures against a background of very low chronic exposure, but another may have had relatively constant, modestly elevated exposure. Some neuropsychological deficits may result primarily from chronic exposure, and others may be acute pharmacologic effects of recent exposures (Winneke, Beginn, Ewert, Havestadt, Kraemer, Krause, Thron, & Wagner, 1985).

Under the plausible hypothesis that stage of brain development at the time of exposure determines the neuropsychological domain in which lead toxicity is expressed, heterogeneity in the exposure profiles of children in a cohort will produce heterogeneity in neuropsychological presentation. Under these circumstances, any lead effects may be manifested as small differences on tests that integrate performance over a broad range of domains (e.g., IQ tests). The heterogeneity in presentation might be interpreted to mean that lead effects are idiopathic. A hypothesis that should be considered, however, is that differences in temporal features of exposure profiles are responsible for some portion of the heterogeneity.

The most systematic attempt to link different patterns of exposure to different patterns of expression was a study by Shaheen (1984) of 18 lead-poisoned children and controls matched for sex, age, race, socioeconomic status, and community of residence. Because the children were clinically lead poisoned, unusually detailed blood lead histories were available and children could be classified according to the assumed timing of lead poisoning: early (before age 2), middle (between ages 2 and 3), and late (after age 3). Arguing on the basis of Luria's model that language depends on earlier-maturing secondary cortical areas and visuo-spatial skills on tertiary areas, Shaheen hypothesized that the problems of children poisoned early should primarily involve language skills but the problems of children poisoned later should primarily involve spatial-symbolic skills. Indeed, her data generally supported this hypothesis, suggesting that taking account of age at critical exposure, information that is unavailable in most studies, may bring some coherence to the confusing data presently available on the specific neuropsychological effects of lead. In developmental toxicity assessments using animals, many dosing regimens are used (Nelson, 1991), and the influence of lead-dosing regimen on behavioral outcome is evident in both primates (Rice, 1992b) and rodents (Cory-Slechta, 1990). The exposure profiles of the children participating in the prospective lead studies differ in many ways (e.g., level of prenatal exposure, slope and timing of postnatal increase in blood lead). The pharmacokinetic implications of these differences support study-specific predictions about the patterns of associations that should be observed in the various studies (Mushak, 1993).

Future studies must include much more detailed and comprehensive assessments of body lead burden. Ideally, this approach will include longitudinal measurements of lead concentration in multiple body pools. The search to understand the brain–behavior relationships underlying lead neurotoxicity would be advanced considerably if we had a validated biokinetic model that estimated lead at the critical target organ for neurotoxicity, the brain.

Whenever the neuropsychological toxicity of any chemical is under investigation, the strategy for determining exposure must take into account the specific biokinetic characteristics of the compound (Dietrich & Bellinger, 1994). For lipophilic substances such as methylmercury or polychlorinated biphenyls (PCBs), levels in blood serum, hair, adipose tissue aspirates, or breast milk may be useful indices of internal exposure. These media are not as useful for inorganic compounds (e.g., the chemical form of lead that is the greatest worry on a population basis). In studying environmental PCBs, an investigator must contend with the possibility that these complex mixtures of 209 distinct congeners differ greatly in toxicity (Birnbaum, 1993). Compounds of interest may also be contaminated to varying degrees by other neurotoxic compounds. For example, in the *Yu-Cheng* episode of rice oil poisoning in Taiwan (Rogan, Gladen, Hung, Koong, Shih, Taylor, Wu, Yang, Ragan, & Hsu, 1988), the presence of highly toxic dibenzofurans in the oil precluded definitive identification of PCBs as the agent responsible for the neurodevelopmental problems of the exposed children. Compounds with short biological residence times, such as organophosphate pesticides and organic solvents, may allow few options for direct assessment of body burden following cessation of exposure. In such cases, exposure must generally be classified by indirect measures such as duration of residence in a contaminated area, distance of residence from the source of contamination, or amount of contaminated foodstuffs consumed.

Lead-Environment Interactions

Attempts to interpret the literature on lead often appear to rest on the assumption that all studies are equivalent and should arrive at the same answer. In the preceding section we discuss how differences in exposure patterns may contribute to differences in study findings. Other study differences also may be important. In trying to resolve interstudy inconsistencies, the first step taken by investigators working with animal models is to consider differences in the "experimental systems" used. Conversely, the almost exclusive focus of efforts to reconcile conflicting data in epidemiologic lead studies is differences in statistical modeling and control of confounding bias. The cohorts under prospective study differ in demographic characteristics, hence in distribution of developmental risks other than lead (e.g., mean maternal IQs in the Boston and Cleveland cohorts differ by 45 points). These can be viewed as analogous to differences in genotype, animal housing and handling practices, or behavioral testing history. The behavioral pharmacology literature has many examples of drug toxicity depending on an animal's experience within the environment in which the drug is administered (MacPhail, 1990). The experimental procedures an animal has undergone, analogous to differences in life experiences or rearing environment, can alter the form or magnitude of lead-associated behavioral deficits in primates (Rice, 1992c). Other studies show that lead effects can be masked by co-occurring exposures, such as the parasite *toxocara canis* (Dolinsky, Burright, Donovick, Glickman, Babish, Summers, & Cypess, 1981) or cadmium (Nation, Grover, Bratton, & Salinas, 1990). Finally, the hormonal effects of important experiences, such as confinement, can affect lead metabolism, stimulating mobilization from deep body pools (Bushnell, Shelton, & Bowman, 1979).

As we saw earlier, lead-exposed primates consistently demonstrate marked individual variability in behavioral impairment. This aspect of performance is considered a potentially important index of toxicity in animal studies; that is, an endpoint in itself (Weiss, 1988). In human studies it tends to be considered statistical "noise" that impedes identification of between-group differences in mean performance. Clinicians have long recognized substantial variation in the likelihood that an individual will display clinical signs of lead toxicity at a given blood lead level (U.S. EPA, 1986a). Apart from investigations of sociodemographic factors, the bases for individual differences in human susceptibility have been the object of more speculation than study. Two decades ago, it was hypothesized that African-American children are more vulnerable to lead than Caucasian children because of higher prevalence of a deficiency in the enzyme glucose-6-phosphate dehydrogenase (McIntire & Angle, 1972). Another hypothesis based on genetic variation was advanced by Wetmur, Lehnert, & Desnick (1991), proposing that individuals expressing a specific allele (1-2 or 2-2) of the heme pathway enzyme amino levulinic acid dehydratase (ALA-D) tend to have higher blood-lead levels than individuals expressing the more common variant (1-1), perhaps reflecting greater vulnerability. In a later section, we describe some preliminary work exploring this possibility.

Mechanisms of Lead Neurotoxicity

Knowledge of or hypotheses about the mechanism underlying a neurotoxic insult or the site of the resulting lesion can sometimes guide attempts to characterize the primary neuropsychological effect of an exposure or event (e.g., phenylketonuria and damage to the dopaminergic system of the prefrontal cortex; Smith, Kates, & Vriezen, 1993). Although considerable effort has been invested in searching for the specific site(s) and mechanism(s) of lead neurotoxicity, there is "no unifying hypothesis of the fundamental neurobiological mechanisms of lead toxicity" (Silbergeld, 1992a, p. 90). Lead's effects are legion and apparent in many organ systems. One reason is the very general level at which lead poisons physiologic processes. It binds to sulfhydryl groups on enzyme proteins, altering their molecular conformation, hence their biological activity. One well-characterized effect of lead is its interference with various steps in the heme biosynthetic pathway. Because hemoproteins are involved in many systems, any perturbation in their production produces a cascade of effects. In the blood-forming system oxygen transport is impaired, in the nervous system cellular energetics are impaired, in the kidney and endocrine systems calcium metabolism is impaired, and in the liver detoxification processes are impaired.

Silbergeld (1992b) argues that several distinct mechanisms of lead neurotoxicity are likely. It may be a "neurodevelopmental toxicant," interfering with the development of cell:cell connections and thus neuronal cytoarchitecture. It also may be a "neuropharmacological toxicant," interfering with ionic mechanisms of cell:cell interactions, i.e., neurotransmission between and within neurons.

The multiple levels of mechanism may work in concert. Because lead is not a general cytotoxin, at least at the lower body burdens of greatest worry at the population level, it does not reduce the number of neurons although it may reduce the number of synaptic connections (McCauley, Bull, Tonti, Lutkenhoff, Meister, Doerger, & Stober, 1982). Goldstein (1990, 1992) proposes that lead may disrupt the activity- or experience-driven selective pruning of synapses that "overgrow" in the early postnatal period (Oppenheim, 1991). By increasing the tonic release of neurotransmitter (i.e., without depolarization of the postsynaptic cell), lead may alter the trophic environment and thus the likelihood that "useful" synapses will survive or that incorrectly targeted neuronal projections will be eliminated. The result would be a nervous system with an appropriate number of cells and connections and one without gross morphological pathology but, Goldstein says, one "with poorly chosen connections" in which "systems matching" (O'Leary, 1987) has failed. This condition ultimately could be expressed as subtle impairments in learning and behavior. Several lines of evidence support aspects of this hypothesis. Regan and colleagues show that lead at low dose disrupts the functioning of rat cerebellar neural cell adhesion molecule, a morphoregulator that directs fiber outgrowth and routing (Cookman, King, & Regan, 1987; Regan, 1989). Lead also affects differentiation of glial cells and thus their function as pathway or trophic supports for establishing neuronal connections (Cookman, Hemmens, Keane, King, & Regan, 1988; Stark, Wolff, & Korbmacher, 1992; Tiffany-Castiglioni, Sierra, Wu, & Rowles, 1989).

Abundant evidence demonstrates that lead is a neuropharmacologic toxicant affecting neurotransmission and signal transduction (Audesirk, 1985). Many of these effects are the result of lead's interference with calcium metabolism (i.e., binding, storage, release). Given the importance of calcium in regulating the neuronal environment, the sensitivity of calcium and calcium-regulated processes to lead provides a plausible mechanism (or set of mechanisms) for lead neurotoxicity (Bondy, 1989; Kennedy, 1989; Pounds & Rosen, 1988). The interactions between lead and calcium take various forms, with lead preventing calcium from reaching receptor sites, disturbing intracellular and extracellular calcium distribution, and replacing calcium in its regulatory roles (Goldstein, 1992). For instance, protein kinase C, a second messenger, is exquisitely sensitive to lead, responding at picomolar concentrations (Markovac & Goldstein, 1988). A possible basis for lead's long-term effects on cognition is suggested by lead's ability to block NMDA receptors at glutamate synapses in rat hippocampal pyramidal cells (Alkondon, Costa, Radhakrishnan, Aronstam, & Albuquerque, 1990). Protein kinase C modulates NMDA receptor currents and thus may induce long-term potentiation, hypothesized to be the neural basis for learning and memory (Ben-Ari, Aniksztejn, & Bregestovski, 1992). The "neuropharmacologic" and "neurodevelopmental" mechanisms of lead neurotoxicity may work together. For instance, by modulating synaptic activity, calcium ions also affect adhesive interactions and thus synaptic efficiency (Schubert, 1991).

Although the mechanism(s) of low-level lead effects is uncertain, that of high-level effects is most likely to involve disturbances in the homeostatic functions served by the endothelial cells in microvessels that constitute the blood–brain barrier. The breakdown in their barrier functions may be mediated by lead effects on supporting astrocytes, producing the classic clinical signs of lead poisoning, including brain edema and increased intracranial pressure (Goldstein, 1992). Goldstein speculates that lead effects on energy-dependent trophic functions of the blood–brain barrier, such as the active pumping of potassium and other ions, amino acids, and neurotransmitters, also may contribute to the putative effects of low levels of lead on neural organization during critical periods of development. Evidence of lead-induced leakage of plasma proteins across the blood–brain barrier in the absence of edema is consistent with this hypothesis (Sundstrom, Muntzing, Kalimo, & Sourander, 1985).

Clearly, lead has myriad effects on biological systems, from the molecular to whole organ-system level, some of which may ultimately be expressed as behavioral toxicity. Probably no one, perhaps not even a primary neurobiological effect is responsible. Accordingly, lead almost certainly has no one "behavioral signature." The form in which toxicity is expressed can be expected to vary with the age at which an organism is exposed, the age at which it is tested, the task on which it is tested, the environment in which testing occurs, the life experiences of the organism both prior to and after exposure (including coexposures), and the characteristics of the exposure (dose, timing, duration). Because very few of these factors have been examined for their influence on outcome, it is not terribly surprising that little progress has been achieved in characterizing brain–behavior relationships. What is surprising is the degree of overall consistency across studies in the mere presence of lead-associated performance decrements on global indices of function.

In trying to understand why progress has been so slow, we must recognize that the primary goal in most studies on low-level lead toxicity has been to answer a question that primarily interests the public-health community: "Can *any* differences be identified in the performance of children with lead exposures that are in the upper reaches of the range currently considered to be 'normal'?" Typically the specific performance difference associated with increased exposure has been of less interest than the fact of the difference. Because the purpose was to provide an empirical basis for public-policy formulation, it also has been necessary to make this difference, whatever it is, understandable and easily communicated to and accepted by those without scientific training. Not surprisingly, IQ-like measures have been chosen as the major endpoints. Everyone thinks he or she knows what IQ is, responds to its mystique, and knows that higher is better. Public-health officials are much more likely to be moved to action by pollutant-related effects on IQ than by effects on fixed-interval schedules of reinforcement or an experimental laboratory test which may be of great theoretical interest and promise but which is not considered well validated. Because IQ change can be monetized, this endpoint also lends itself nicely to cost–benefit computations, permitting straightforward comparisons of the economic implications of alternative regulatory proposals (e.g., U.S. EPA, 1986b).

Another reason that IQ measures have been the primary focus of most studies relates to their strong psychometric properties. Because the goal in most studies has been to identify the "lowest observed effect level" (LOEL), the sampling frames have been designed to recruit study cohorts with lead levels at or below the current screening targets. Any lead effect in such a cohort will necessarily be subtle, requiring the most sensitive assessments. Many of the neuropsychological tests used in clinical settings may simply not be as sensitive as IQ tests to small performance variations within the normal range. To maximize information yield and communicability while minimizing cost, most investigators have relied on IQ tests, which yield a little information about a broad range of domains in a relatively brief time.

The goals and methods of these investigations differ from those of an investigation in which lead-exposed children are studied as a means to a neuropsychological end (i.e., as a model system for investigating the effect of a neurotoxicant on brain–behavior relationships). The study by Shaheen (1984) described earlier is a rare example of an effort to look beyond IQ scores to understand how and why performance by lead-exposed children on IQ tests differs from that of peers with lesser exposures. In public-health–oriented epidemiological studies, the investigation of lead tends to be viewed solely as an end in itself. It is not necessary to understand how toxicity works to justify public-health action. The pathogenesis of toxic shock syndrome was still being studied long after removal of a brand of tampon from the marketplace just about eliminated incident cases (Centers for Disease Control, 1981; Langmuir, 1982). Similarly, the spread of cholera in nineteenth-century London was halted by removing the handle from the Broad Street water pump, long before the *vibrio* bacillus was identified as the pathogen (Hill, 1953). Of course understanding the mechanism may make the rationale for action more compelling and may be helpful in designing the most effective plan.

It seems evident that studies seeking to characterize underlying behavioral pathology may require different design strategies than studies seeking to define dose-response or dose-effect relationships. An investigator seeking such information has two choices: (1) devise new tests of greater sensitivity but which will perforce enjoy less widespread use and acceptance, or (2) continue to use stock tests but with them study children with exposures well above those suspected of defining LOELs, in whom any toxicant-associated effects may be large enough to be apparent despite limited sensitivity. Adopting the latter approach requires assuming, however, that the performance decrements produced by lower exposures share the same neuropsychological basis as deficits produced by higher exposures. This is the strategy followed by Faust and Brown (1987), who administered a broad-based battery of psychometric and clinical tests based on Luria's model to 15 lead-exposed children and matched controls (the highest recorded blood lead levels of the exposed group averaged 52 µg/dL). The lower overall performance of the exposed children relative to their controls was due to consistently lower scores on most tests administered rather than to large differences in specific areas. Faust and Brown concluded that "a specific pattern of cognitive deficit" was not apparent, although the small sample size seriously limited the possibility of detecting any pattern amid the substantial heterogeneity in the performance of the exposed group.

Our group (Bellinger, Hu, Titlebaum, & Needleman, 1994) also adopted this approach, following up in young adulthood individuals who had participated as first- and second-graders in a study by Needleman et al. (1979). The concentration of lead in the dentin of shed deciduous teeth, which averaged about 14 micrograms per gram (μg/g or parts per million), served as one exposure index. By comparison, the mean concentration in a population-based cohort in the Boston area about a decade later was only 3 μg/g (Leviton, Bellinger, Allred, Rabinowitz, Needleman, & Schoenbaum, 1993). Based on childhood screening results available for some children, the blood-lead range probably was from 15 to 50 μg/dL. We also measured the concentration of lead in bone (midshaft left tibia and left patella) by K-X-ray-fluorescence. Lead concentrations in both teeth and bone are biologic markers of past exposure (Rosen, 1988).

Previous follow-up assessments indicated that children with higher dentin lead levels had slightly lower IQs (4 points), slower reaction time, auditory-linguistic and reading-performance deficits, poorer classroom behavior, and slower school progress (Bellinger, Needleman, Bromfield, & Mintz, 1984; Needleman, Gunnoe, Leviton, Reed, Peresie, Maher, & Barrett, 1979; Needleman, Schell, Bellinger, Leviton, & Allred, 1990). In planning an additional follow-up study of these young adults, we considered several general hypotheses about possible bases for these performance deficits. Among the many possibilities are these: (1) general, across-the-board impairment of cognition or its output (i.e., generalized performance decrement); (2) the joint effect of various independent impairments (i.e., lead may have many separate targets in the nervous system); or (3) impairment of a small set of key functions that contribute to performance in many cognitive domains. In the interest of parsimony, we pursued the latter hypothesis, seeking to identify a function which underlies performance on many psychometric and neuropsychological tests and which may represent the primary "neuropsychological lesion" produced by lead. Based on previous human and animal work, the obvious candidate for first consideration is "attention." In most lead studies, attention has been operationalized simply as performance on simple or choice reaction-time tasks or as teacher or parent ratings of distractibility, impulsivity, or impersistence. In an effort to go beyond this conceptualization, we selected the multielement model of attention and information processing developed by Mirsky and colleagues at NIMH, including the empirically derived battery of tests purported to tap elements of the hypothesized model (Mirsky, Anthony, Duncan, Ahearn, & Kellam, 1991). In factor analyzing adults' and children's performance on tests usually considered to assess some aspect of attention, they consistently

Table 2.2. Tests comprising the attention battery.

ENCODE
Digit-span subtest of the WAIS-R
Arithmetic subtest of the WAIS-R
FOCUS-EXECUTE
Talland Letter Cancellation (total number correct in 6 sets of trials, 2 each in which target was capital letters, double spaces, or both)
Stroop Color-Word Interference Test (time needed to complete the Color and Color-Word Interference trials)
Digit-symbol subtest of the WAIS-R
Trail-Making Test (time needed to complete Parts A and B)
SUSTAIN
Visual Continuous Performance Test (number of correct responses, number of commission errors, reaction time for correct responses)
SHIFT
Wisconsin Card Sorting Test (number of errors) (other scores recorded include the number of correct responses, number of categories achieved, number of perseverative errors)

Source: Developed by Mirsky et al. (1991).

identified four elements of this construct: (1) encode ("... the sequential registration, recall, and mental manipulation of numeric information," p. 118); (2) focus-execute ("... the ability to select target information from an array for enhanced processing," p. 111); (3) sustain ("... the capacity to maintain focus and alertness over time, or vigilance," p. 112); and (4) shift ("... the ability to change attentive focus in a flexible and adaptive manner," p. 112). Table 2.2 lists the tests in the battery and the factors to which they pertain.

The battery was administered to seventy-nine 19- and 20-year-olds. Multivariate regression analyses were carried out in which the test scores contributing to each of the four components of attention were treated as joint dependent variables and examined in relation to the concentration of lead in dentin and bone. Adjustment was made for parent IQ, maternal age, maternal education, family social class, sex, birth order, and current use of cigarettes, illicit drugs, and alcohol.

Higher dentin lead levels were associated with significantly lower covariate-adjusted scores on the Focus-Execute and Shift components of attention and to scores on many of the individual tests contributing to these factors. Scores on most tests changed in a dose-dependent fashion (Table 2.3). In addition to being related to the number of errors on the Wisconsin Card Sorting Test, dentin lead level was inversely related to the number of categories achieved and positively associated with the number of perseverative responses.

Tibia lead levels were inversely related to performance on the Focus-Execute component of attention, but to no other. Patella lead levels were not related to any of the four components. These findings should be

Table 2.3. Adjusted scores on tests in attention battery for children, classified by dentin lead quartile.

	Dentin Lead Quartile			
	1	2	3	4
Attention factor	(2.9–5.9)	(6.0–8.7)	(8.8–19.8)	(19.9–51.8)
ENCODE				
Digit span	11.8 (0.6)[a]	11.4 (0.6)	10.5 (0.7)	10.3 (0.6)
Arithmetic	11.2 (0.5)	11.5 (0.5)	11.4 (0.6)	11.0 (0.5)
FOCUS-EXECUTE				
Digit symbol	11.5 (0.7)	11.0 (0.7)	10.2 (0.8)	9.8 (0.7)
Cancellation	305.1 (15.2)	288.3 (15.0)	296.4 (16.4)	253.0 (15.2)
Trials A	26.0 (2.3)	26.7 (2.2)	30.7 (2.4)	30.5 (2.3)
Trials B	54.6 (4.8)	54.2 (4.7)	60.3 (5.2)	72.1 (4.8)
Stroop-Color	51.9 (3.4)	56.3 (3.3)	56.3 (3.7)	65.4 (3.4)
Stroop-Color/Word	103.3 (8.1)	115.7 (7.6)	126.5 (8.4)	124.7 (7.7)
SUSTAIN (CPT)				
No. correct	98.0 (1.0)	97.6 (1.1)	96.9 (1.1)	94.6 (1.1)
No. commission errors	0.2 (0.1)	0.1 (0.1)	0.3 (0.1)	0.2 (0.1)
Reaction time	361.2 (16.5)	374.1 (17.3)	370.7 (17.9)	385.0 (17.1)
SHIFT (Wisconsin Card Sorting Test)				
No. errors	14.1 (3.8)	22.9 (3.7)	20.9 (4.1)	32.2 (3.7)
No. correct	70.5 (2.9)	72.7 (2.8)	74.5 (3.1)	71.4 (2.9)
No. categories	6.1 (0.3)	5.6 (0.3)	5.3 (0.3)	4.9 (0.3)
No. perseverative errors	8.1 (2.2)	12.8 (2.2)	12.4 (2.4)	17.3 (2.2)

mean ± standard error.
Source: Adapted from Bellinger et al. (1994).

interpreted cautiously because of the substantial uncertainty presently associated with the bone lead measurements. It is noteworthy, however, that tibia consists of dense cortical bone with a relatively slow turnover rate (~2.5% per year) but the patella (kneecap) consists of spongy trabecular bone, which has a faster turnover rate (~10% per year) (Grandjean, 1988). In adulthood, lead concentration in cortical bone may provide a better index of childhood lead exposure than does the lead concentration in the more dynamic trabecular bone.

In this study we also explored the contribution of genetic variation to variability in neuropsychological performance. Using venous blood samples, we characterized the ALA-D isozyme phenotypes of the young adults. As expected, most expressed the 1-1 allele. Five of the 72 who contributed blood samples expressed the 1-2 allele. No one expressed the 2-2 allele. Adjusting for differences in dentin lead levels, the 5 individuals with the 1-2 allele achieved better scores than the individuals with the 1-1 allele on nearly every test administered. This finding clearly needs to be confirmed in a larger sample, but it suggests that genetic variability in biochemical systems involved in metabolizing lead may account for some of the individual variability in the effect of lead on neuropsychological performance. Recent work also has identified lead-binding proteins in various organ systems, including the brain, which may affect the transport and ultimate disposition of lead in the CNS (Goering, Mistry, & Fowler, 1986). The present strategy of using the concentration of lead in a peripheral tissue as the sole basis for classifying individuals' exposure (and thus assuming that all individuals with a specific lead level are equally vulnerable) clearly involves substantial risk of misclassification. The search for specific neuropsychological target(s) of lead will almost certainly be more successful once biologic markers of vulnerability are identified and taken into account. Such integration of molecular epidemiology and neuropsychology is an exciting new direction in understanding brain–behavior relationships.

These findings provide some clues as to the bases of lead-associated performance differences on global indices. They suggest that one target, at least at higher levels of exposure, may be executive or regulatory functions (the ability to identify goals and to execute plans to achieve them). The behaviors of the more highly exposed children bear striking similarities to those of lead-dosed primates, who perform poorly on discrimination-reversal tasks and learning set formation (cf. number of errors on the WCST) (Rice, 1992a). More highly exposed monkeys also show marked perseveration on spatial delayed-alternation tasks and delayed match-to-sample tasks (cf. perseveration errors on the WCST), as well as markedly diminished performance in the presence of irrelevant or distracting cues on discrimination-reversal tasks (cf. slower performance on the Stroop Test and letter cancelation task).

Conclusion

With the recognition that the target organ most sensitive to environmental toxicants may be the nervous system (Kilburn, 1989) has come increasing acceptance of behavior and development as important components in toxicity assessment (Russell, Flattau, & Pope, 1990). Also gaining favor is the view that some portion of psychiatric and neurological morbidity is attributable to chemical exposures (Weiss, 1985). For no pollutant has this view been developed as extensively as it has for lead. Indeed, among the recommendations in the most recent lead statement by the Committee on Environmental Hazards of the American Academy of Pediatrics is: "Lead poisoning should be considered in the evaluation of the following disorders, either because the lead may cause these disorders or because the conditions may be associated with increased lead ingestion: developmental delay, learning disabilities, behavior disorder, autism, convulsions, iron deficiency anemia, intestinal parasitic infections, speech and hearing deficits, encephalopathy, recurrent vomiting, and recurrent abdominal pain" (AAP, 1993, p. 181).

Neuropsychologists are likely to become increasingly involved in evaluating and managing children exposed to environmental pollutants, as well as in research to characterize the CNS influence of such compounds more precisely. This change will require greater appreciation for concepts and methods that generally do not arise in the neuropsychological study of other medical conditions and events. Among the factors to consider are the unique toxicokinetics of specified compounds including chemical speciation (organic vs. inorganic forms), routes and patterns of exposure that may affect the form and severity of toxicity, and the complex web of caregiving factors that may mask, mimic, exacerbate, or otherwise affect the manner in which toxicity is expressed. Despite all the research on childhood lead poisoning conducted over the past 50 years, the remaining sketchiness in our understanding of many aspects of lead's influence on neuropsychological functioning bears witness to the difficulty of discerning clear answers.

Acknowledgments. The research conducted by our group was supported by NIH grants HD08945, HD17407, HD25114, ES04095, ES00138 (a Research Career Development Award), and HD18655 (A Mental Retardation Research Center grant). Other members of the research team have included Herbert L. Needleman, M.D., Alan Leviton, M.D., Michael Rabinowitz, Ph.D., Karen Stiles, Ph.D., Jone Sloman, Ph.D., Elizabeth Allred, M.S., Christine Waternaux, Ph.D., and Molly Nichols, B.S.

References

Achenbach, T., Howell, C., Aoki, M., & Rauh, V. (1993). Nine-year outcome of the Vermont Intervention Program for low birth weight infants. *Pediatrics, 91,* 45–55.

Alkondon M., Costa, A., Radhakrishnan, V., Aronstam, R., & Albuquerque, E. (1990). Selective blockade of NMDA-activated channel currents may be implicated in learning deficits caused by lead. *FEBS Letters, 261,* 124–130.

American Academy of Pediatrics Committee on Environmental Health. (1993). Lead poisoning: From screening to primary prevention. *Pediatrics, 92,* 176–183.

Annest, J., Pirkle, J., Makuc, D., Neese, J., Bayse, D., & Kovar, M. (1983). Chronological trend in blood lead levels between 1986 and 1980. *New England Journal of Medicine, 308,* 1373–1377.

Audesirk, G. (1985). Effects of lead exposure on the physiology of neurons. *Progress in Neurobiology, 24,* 199–231.

Aylward, G. (1992). The relationship between environmental risk and developmental outcome. *Journal of Developmental and Behavioral Pediatrics, 13,* 222–229.

Aylward, G. (1993). Perinatal asphyxia: Effects of biologic and environmental risks. *Clinics in Perinatology, 20,* 433–449.

Baghurst, P., McMichael, A., Wigg, N., Vimpani, G., Robertson, E., Roberts, R., & Tong, S-L. (1992). Environmental exposure to lead and children's intelligence at the age of seven years. *New England Journal of Medicine, 327,* 1279–1284.

Bellinger, D., Needleman, H., Bromfield, R., & Mintz, M. (1984). A follow-up study of the academic attainment and classroom behavior of children with elevated dentine lead levels. *Biological Trace Element Research, 6,* 207–223.

Bellinger, D., Needleman, H., Leviton, A., Waternaux, C., Rabinowitz, M., & Nichols, M. (1984). Early sensory-motor development and prenatal exposure to lead. *Neurobehavioral Toxicology and Teratology, 6,* 387–402.

Bellinger, D., Leviton, A., Waternaux, C., & Allred, E. (1985). Methodological issues in modeling the relationship between low-level lead exposure and infant development: Examples from the Boston Lead Study. *Environmental Research, 38,* 119–129.

Bellinger, D., Leviton, A., Needleman, H., Waternaux, C., & Rabinowitz, M. (1986). Low-level lead exposure and infant development in the first year. *Neurobehavioral Toxicology and Teratology, 8,* 151–161.

Bellinger, D., Leviton, A., Rabinowitz, M., Needleman, H., & Waternaux, C. (1986). Correlates of low-level lead exposure in urban children at two years of age. *Pediatrics, 77,* 826–833.

Bellinger, D., Leviton, A., Waternaux, C., Needleman, H., & Rabinowitz, M. (1987). Longitudinal analyses of pre- and postnatal lead exposure and early cognitive development. *New England Journal of Medicine, 316,* 1037–1043.

Bellinger, D., Leviton, A., Waternaux, C., Needleman, H., & Rabinowitz, M. (1988). Low-level lead exposure, social class, and infant development. *Neurotoxicology and Teratology, 10,* 497–503.

Bellinger, D., Leviton, A., & Waternaux, C. (1989). Lead, IQ, and social class. *International Journal of Epidemiology, 18,* 180–185.

Bellinger, D., Leviton, A., Waternaux, C., Needleman, H., & Rabinowitz, M. (1989). Low-level lead exposure and early development in socioeconomically advantaged urban infants. In M. Smith, L. Grant, & A. Sors (Eds.), *Lead Exposure and Child Development: An International Assessment* (pp. 345–356). Dordrecht: Kluwer Academic Publishers.

Bellinger, D., Leviton, A., & Sloman, J. (1990). Antecedents and correlates of improved cognitive performance in children exposed in utero to low levels of lead. *Environmental Health Perspectives, 89,* 5–11.

Bellinger, D., Sloman, J., Leviton, A., Rabinowitz, M., Needleman, H., & Waternaux, C. (1991). Low-level lead exposure and children's cognitive function in the preschool years. *Pediatrics, 87,* 219–227.

Bellinger, D., & Needleman, H. (1992). Neurodevelopmental effects of low-level lead exposure in children. In H. Needleman (Ed.), *Human Lead Exposure* (pp. 191–208). Boca Raton: CRC Press.

Bellinger, D., Stiles, K., & Needleman, H. (1992). Low-level lead exposure, intelligence, and academic achievement: A long-term follow-up study. *Pediatrics, 90,* 855–861.

Bellinger, D., & Stiles, K. (1993). Epidemiologic approaches to assessing the developmental neurotoxicity of lead. *NeuroToxicology, 14,* 151–160.

Bellinger, D., & Dietrich, K. (in press). Recent studies of lead and neurobehavioral development in children. *Occupational Medicine: State of the Art Reviews.*

Bellinger, D., Hu, H., Titlebaum, L., & Needleman, H. (1992). Attentional correlates of dentin and bone lead levels in adolescents. *Archives of Environmental Health*, *49*, 98–105.

Ben-Ari, Y., Aniksztejn, L., & Bregestovski, P. (1992). Protein kinase C modulation of NMDA currents: An important link for LTP induction. *Trends in Neuroscience, 15,* 333–339.

Bergomi, M., Borella, P., Fantuzzi, G., Vivoli, G., Sturloni, N., Cavazzuti, G., Tampieri, A., & Tartoni, P. (1989). Relationship between lead exposure indicators and neuropsychological performance in children. *Developmental Medicine and Child Neurology, 31,* 181–190.

Birnbaum, L. (1993). Pharmacokinetics of PCBs. In U.S. Environmental Protection Agency, *Workshop Report on Developmental Neurotoxic Effects Associated with Exposure to PCBs* (pp. 2–7 to 2–10). EPA/630/R-92/004.

Bondy, S. (1989). Intracellular calcium and neurotoxic events. *Neurotoxicology and Teratology, 11,* 527–531.

Burbacher, T., Rodier, P., & Weiss, B. (1990). Methylmercury developmental neurotoxicity: A comparison of effects in humans and animals. *Neurotoxicology and Teratology, 12,* 191–202.

Bushnell, P., Shelton, S., & Bowman, R. (1979). Elevation of blood lead concentration by confinement in the rhesus monkey. *Bulletin of Environmental Contamination and Toxicology, 22,* 819–826.

Byers, R., & Lord, E. (1943). Late effects of lead poisoning on mental development. *American Journal of Diseases of Children, 66,* 471–494.

Centers for Disease Control. (1981). Toxic-shock syndrome—United States, 1970–1980. *Morbidity and Mortality Weekly Report, 30,* 25–28.

Centers for Disease Control. (1991). *Preventing Lead Poisoning in Young Children: A Statement by the Centers for Disease Control.* U.S. Department of Health and Human Services.

Cookman, G., King, W., & Regan, C. (1987). Chronic low-level lead exposure impairs embryonic to adult conversion of the neural cell adhesion molecule. *Journal of Neurochemistry, 49,* 399–403.

Cookman, G., Hemmens, S., Keane, G., King, W., & Regan, C. (1988). Chronic low level-lead exposure precociously induces rat glial development in vitro and in vivo. *Neuroscience Letters, 86,* 33–37.

Cooney, G., Bell, A., McBride, W., & Carter, C. (1989a). Low-level exposures to lead: The Sydney Lead Study. *Developmental Medicine and Child Neurology, 31,* 640–649.

Cooney, G., Bell, A., McBride, W., & Carter, C. (1989b). Neurobehavioral consequences of prenatal low level exposure to lead. *Neurotoxicology and Teratology, 11,* 95–104.

Cory-Slechta, D. (1990). Exposure duration modifies the effects of low level lead on fixed-interval performance. *NeuroToxicology, 11,* 427–442.

Davies, J. (1990). Neurotoxic concerns of human pesticide exposures. *American Journal of Industrial Medicine, 18,* 327–331.

Dietrich, K., Krafft, K., Bornschein, R., Hammond, P., Berger, O., Succop, P., & Bier, M. (1987). Low-level fetal lead exposure effect on neurobehavioral development in early infancy. *Pediatrics, 80,* 721–730.

Dietrich, K., Succop, P., Bornschein, R., Krafft, K., Berger, O., Hammond, P., & Buncher, R. (1990). Lead exposure and neurobehavioral development in later infancy. *Environmental Health Perspectives, 89,* 13–19.

Dietrich, K., Succop, P., Berger, O., Hammond, P., & Bornschein, R. (1991). Lead exposure and the cognitive development of urban preschool children: The Cincinnati Lead Study cohort at age 4 years. *Neurotoxicology and Teratology, 13,* 203–211.

Dietrich, K., Succop, P., Berger, O., & Keith, R. (1992). Lead exposure and the central auditory processing abilities and cognitive development of urban children: The Cincinnati Lead Study cohort at age 5 years. *Neurotoxicology and Teratology, 14,* 51–56.

Dietrich, K., Berger, O., & Succop, P. (1993a). Lead exposure and the motor developmental status of urban six-year-old children in the Cincinnati Prospective Study. *Pediatrics, 91,* 301–307.

Dietrich, K., Berger, O., Succop, P., & Hammond, P. (1993b). The developmental consequences of low to moderate prenatal and postnatal lead exposure: Intellectual attainment in the Cincinnati Lead Study cohort following school entry. *Neurotoxicology and Teratology, 15,* 37–44.

Dietrich, K., & Bellinger, D. (1994). Assessment of neurobehavioral development in studies of the effects of fetal exposures to environmental agents. In H. Needleman & D. Bellinger (Eds.), *Prenatal Exposure to Environmental Toxicants: Developmental Consequences* (pp. 57–85). Baltimore: Johns Hopkins Press.

Dolinsky, Z., Burright, R., Donovick, P., Glickman, L., Babish, J., Summers, B., & Cypess, R. (1981). Behavioral effects of lead and *toxocara canis* in mice. *Science, 213,* 1142–1144.

Ernhart, C., Landa, B., & Schell, N. (1981). Subclinical levels of lead and developmental deficit: A multivariate follow-up reassessment. *Pediatrics, 67,* 911–919.

Ernhart, C., Morrow-Tlucak, M., Marler, M., & Wolf, A. (1987). Low-level lead exposure in the prenatal and early preschool periods: Early preschool development. *Neurotoxicology and Teratology, 9,* 259–270.

Ernhart, C., Morrow-Tlucak, M., Wolf, A., Super, D., & Drotar, D. (1989). Low-level lead exposure in the prenatal and early postnatal periods: Intelligence prior to school entry. *Neurotoxicology and Teratology, 11,* 161–170.

Faust, D., & Brown, J. (1987). Moderately elevated blood lead levels: Effects on neuropsychologic functioning in children. *Pediatrics, 80,* 623–629.

Fergusson, D., Fergusson, J., Horwood, L., & Kinzett, N. (1988). A longitudinal study of dentine lead levels, intelligence, school performance, and behavior: Part II: Dentine lead and cognitive ability. *Journal of Child Psychology and Psychiatry, 29,* 793–809.

Flegal, R., & Smith, D. (1992). Lead levels in preindustrial humans. *New England Journal of Medicine, 326,* 1293–1294.

Gibson, J., Love, W., Hardine, D., Bancroft, P., & Turner, A. (1892). Note on lead poisoning as observed among children in Brisbane. In L. Huxtable (Ed.), *Transactions of the Third Intercolonial Medical Congress of Australia* (pp. 76–83). Sydney: Charles Potter.

Goering, P., Mistry, P., & Fowler, B. (1986). A low molecular weight lead-binding protein in brain attenuates lead inhibition of δ-aminolevulinic acid dehydratase: Comparison with a renal lead-binding protein. *Journal of Pharmacology and Experimental Therapeutics, 237,* 220–225.

Golden, M., & Birns, B. (1983). Social class and infant intelligence. In M. Lewis (Ed.), *Origins of Intelligence: Infancy and Early Childhood*, 2nd Ed. (pp. 347–398). New York: Plenum Press.

Goldstein, G. (1990). Lead poisoning and brain cell function. *Environmental Health Perspectives, 89,* 91–94.

Goldstein, G. (1992). Developmental neurobiology of lead toxicity. In H. Needleman (Ed.), *Human Lead Exposure* (pp. 125–135). Boca Raton, FL: CRC Press.

Goldstein, G., Asbury, A., & Diamond, I. (1974). Pathogenesis of lead encephalopathy: Uptake of lead and reaction of brain capillaries. *Archives of Neurology, 31,* 382–389.

Grandjean, P. (1988). Ancient skeletons as silent witnesses of lead exposures in the past. *CRC Critical Reviews in Toxicology, 19,* 11–21.

Hansen, O., Trillingsgaard, A., Beese, I., Lyngbye, T., & Grandjean, P. (1989). A neuropsychological study of children with elevated dentine lead level: Assessment of the effect of lead in different socio-economic groups. *Neurotoxicology and Teratology, 11,* 205–213.

Harvey, P., Hamlin, M., Kumar, R., & Delves, T. (1984). Blood lead, behavior, and intelligence test performance in pre-school children. *Science of the Total Environment, 40,* 45–60.

Hatzakis, A., Kokkevi, A., Maravelias, C., Katsouyanni, K., Salaminios, F., Kalandidi, A., Koutselinis, A., Stefanis, C., & Trichopoulos, D. (1989). Psychometric intelligence deficits in lead-exposed children. In M. Smith, L. Grant, & A. Sors (Eds.), *Lead Exposure and Child Development: An International Assessment* (pp. 211–223). Dordrecht, Netherlands: Kluwer Academic.

Hill, A. (1953). Observation and experiment. *New England Journal of Medicine, 248,* 995–1001.

Hunter, J., Urbanowicz, M-A., Yule, W., & Lansdown, R. (1985). Automated testing of reaction time and its association with lead in children. *International Archives of Occupational and Environmental Health, 57,* 27–34.

Kennedy, M. (1989). Regulation of neuronal function by calcium. *Trends in Neurosciences, 12,* 417–420.

Kilburn, K. (1989). Is the human nervous system most sensitive to environmental toxins? *Archives of Environmental Health, 44,* 343–344.

Langmuir, A. (1982). Toxic-shock syndrome: An epidemiologist's view. *Journal of Infectious Diseases, 145,* 588–591.

Lansdown, R., Yule, W., Urbanowicz, M-A., & Hunter, J. (1986). The relationship between blood-lead concentrations, intelligence, attainment and behavior in a school population: The second London study. *International Archives of Occupational and Environmental Health, 57,* 225–235.

Leviton, A., Bellinger, D., Allred, E., Rabinowitz, M., Needleman, H., & Schoenbaum, S. (1993). Pre- and postnatal low level lead exposure and children's dysfunction in school. *Environmental Research, 60,* 30–43.

MacPhail, R. (1990). Environmental modulation of neurobehavioral toxicity. In R. Russell, P. Flattau, & A. Pope (Eds.), *Behavioral Measures of Neurotoxicity* (pp. 347–358). Washington, DC, National Academy Press.

Mahaffey, K., Annest, J., Roberts, J., & Murphy, R. (1982). National estimates of blood lead levels: United States 1976–1980. *New England Journal of Medicine, 307,* 573–579.

Marcus, A. (1985). Testing alternative nonlinear kinetic models in compartmental analysis. In J. Eisenfeld & C. Delisi (Eds.), *Mathematics and Computers in Biomedical Applications* (pp. 259–267). Amsterdam: Elsevier.

Marecek, J., Shapiro, I., Burke, A., Katz, S., & Hediger, M. (1983). Low-level lead exposure in childhood influences neuropsychological performance. *Archives of Environmental Health, 38,* 355–359.

Markovac, J., & Goldstein, G. (1988). Picomolar concentrations of lead stimulate brain protein kinase C. *Nature, 334,* 71–73.

McCauley, P., Bull, R., Tonti, A., Lutkenhoff, S., Meister, M., Doerger, J., & Stober, J. (1982). The effect of prenatal and postnatal lead exposure on neonatal synaptogenesis in rat cerebral cortex. *Journal of Toxicology and Environmental Health, 10,* 639–651.

McIntire, M., & Angle, C. (1972). Air lead: Relation to lead in blood of Black school children deficient in glucose-6-phosphate dehydrogenase. *Science, 177,* 520–522.

McMichael, A., Baghurst, P., Wigg, N., Vimpani, G., Robertson, E., & Roberts, R. (1988). Port Pirie Cohort Study: Environmental exposure to lead and children's abilities at the age of four years. *New England Journal of Medicine, 319,* 468–475.

Mills, P., Abbey, D., Beeson, W., & Peterson, F. (1991). Ambient air pollution and cancer in California Seventh-Day Adventists. *Archives of Environmental Health, 46,* 271–280.

Mirsky, A., Anthony, B., Duncan, C., Ahearn, M., & Kellam, S. (1991). Analysis of the elements of attention: A neuropsychological approach. *Neuropsychology Review, 2,* 109–145.

Mushak, P. (1993). New directions in the toxicokinetics of human lead exposure. *Neurotoxicology, 14,* 29–44.

Nation, J., Grover, C., Bratton, G., & Salinas, J. (1990). Behavioral antagonism between lead and cadmium. *Neurotoxicology and Teratology, 12,* 99–104.

National Research Council. (1993). *Measuring Lead Exposure in Infants, Children, and Other Sensitive Populations.* Washington, DC: National Academy Press.

Needleman, H., Gunnoe, C., Leviton, A., Reed, R., Peresie, H., Maher, C., & Barrett, P. (1979). Deficits in psychologic and classroom performance of children with elevated dentine lead levels. *New England Journal of Medicine, 300,* 689–695.

Needleman, H., & Gatsonis, C. (1990). Low-level lead exposure and the IQ of children. *Journal of the American Medical Association, 263,* 673–678.

Needleman, H., Schell, A., Bellinger, D., Leviton, A., & Allred, E. (1990). Long term effects of childhood exposure to lead at low dose: An eleven-year follow-up report. *New England Journal of Medicine, 322,* 83–88.

Needleman, H., & Bellinger, D. (1991). Childhood lead toxicity. *Annual Review of Public Health, 12,* 111–140.

Nelson, B. (1991). Selecting exposure parameters in developmental neurotoxicity assessments. *Neurotoxicology and Teratology, 13,* 569–573.

Nordberg, G., Mahaffey, K., & Fowler, B. (1991). Introduction and summary. International workshop on lead in bone: Implications for dosimetry and toxicology. *Environmental Health Perspectives, 91,* 3–7.

O'Leary, D. (1987). Remodelling of early axonal projections through the selective elimination of neurons and long axon collaterals. In CIBA Foundation Symposium No. 126. *Selective Neuronal Death* (pp. 113–130). New York: John Wiley & Sons.

Oppenheim, R. (1991). Cell death during development of the nervous system. *Annual Review of Neuroscience, 14,* 453–501.

Pounds, J., & Rosen, J. (1988). Cellular Ca^{2+} homeostasis and Ca^{2+}-mediated cell processes as critical targets for toxicant action: Conceptual and methodological pitfalls. *Toxicology and Applied Pharmacology, 94,* 331–341.

Pocock, S., Ashby, D., & Smith, M. (1987). Lead exposure and children's intellectual performance. *International Journal of Epidemiology*, *16*, 57–67.

Raab, G., Thomson, G., Boyd, L., Fulton, M., & Laxen, D. (1990). Blood lead levels, reaction time, inspection time and ability in Edinburgh, Scotland, UK, children. *British Journal of Developmental Psychology, 8,* 101–118.

Rabinowitz, M., & Needleman, H. (1982). Temporal trends in the lead concentrations of umbilical cord blood. *Science, 216,* 1429–1431.

Regan, C. (1989). Lead-impaired neurodevelopment. Mechanisms and threshold values in the rodent. *Neurotoxicology and Teratology, 11,* 533–537.

Rice, D. (1992a). Behavioral impairment produced by developmental lead exposure: Evidence from primate research. In H. Needleman (Ed.), *Human Lead Exposure* (pp. 137–152). Boca Raton, FL: CRC Press.

Rice, D. (1992b). Lead exposure during different developmental periods produces different effects on FI performance in monkeys tested as juveniles and adults. *NeuroToxicology, 13,* 757–770.

Rice, D. (1992c). Behavioral effects of lead in monkeys tested during infancy and adulthood. *Neurotoxicology and Teratology, 14,* 235–245.

Rogan, W., Gladen, B., Hung, K., Koong, S-L., Shih, L-Y., Taylor, J., Wu, Y-C., Yang, D., Ragan, B., & Hsu, C-C. (1988). Congenital poisoning by polychlorinated biphenyls and their contaminants in Taiwan. *Science, 241,* 334–336.

Rosen, J. (1988). The toxicological importance of lead in bone: The evolution and potential uses of bone lead measurements by X-ray fluorescence to evaluate treatment outcomes in moderately lead toxic children. In T. Clarkson, L. Friberg, G. Nordberg, & P. Sager (Eds.), *Biological Monitoring of Toxic Metals* (pp. 603–621). New York: Plenum Publishing.

Rothenberg, S., Lourdes, C., Cansino-Ortiz, S., Perroni-Hernandez, E., de la Torre, P., Neri-Mendez, C., Ortega, P., Hidalgo-Loperena, H., & Svensgaard, D. (1989). Neurobehavioral deficits after low level lead exposure in neonates: The Mexico City Pilot Study. *Neurotoxicology and Teratology, 11,* 85–93.

Rothman, K., & Poole, C. (1988). A strengthening programme for weak associations. *International Journal of Epidemiology, 319,* 955–959.

Russell, R., Flattau, P., & Pope, A. (Eds.) (1990). *Behavioral Measures of Neurotoxicity*. Washington, DC: National Academy Press.

Schubert, D. (1991). The possible role of adhesion in synaptic modification. *Trends in Neurosciences, 14,* 127–130.

Schwartz, J. (1994). Low level lead exposure and children's IQ: A meta analysis and search for a threshold. *Environmental Research*, *65*, 42–55.

Shaheen, S. (1984). Neuromaturation and behavior development: The case of childhood lead poisoning. *Developmental Psychology, 20,* 542–550.

Shapiro, I., & Marecek, J. (1984). Dentine lead concentration as a predictor of neuropsychological functioning in inner-city children. *Biological Trace Element Research, 6,* 69–78.

Silbergeld, E. (1991). Lead in bone: Implications for toxicology during pregnancy and lactation. *Environmental Health Perspectives, 91,* 63–70.

Silbergeld, E. (1992a). Neurological perspective on lead toxicity. In H. Needleman (Ed.), *Human Lead Exposure* (pp. 89–103). Boca Raton, FL: CRC Press.

Silbergeld, E. (1992b). Mechanisms of lead neurotoxicity, or looking beyond the lamppost. *FASEB Journal, 6,* 3201–3206.

Silva, P., Hughes, P., Williams, S., & Faed, W. (1988). Blood lead, intelligence, reading attainment, and behavior in eleven year old children in Dunedin, New Zealand. *Journal of Child Psychology and Psychiatry, 29,* 43–52.

Smith, M., Delves, T., Lansdown, R., Clayton, B., & Graham, P. (1983). The effects of lead exposure on urban children: The Institute of Child Health/Southampton study. *Developmental Medicine and Child Neurology, 25* (Suppl. 47), 1–47.

Smith, M.L., Kates, M., & Vriezen, E. (1993). The development of frontal-lobe functions. In S. Segalowitz & I. Rapin (Eds.), *Handbook of Neuropsychology*, Vol. 7 *Child Neuropsychology* (pp. 309–330). New York: Elsevier.

Stark, M., Wolff, J., & Korbmacher, A. (1992). Modulation of glial cell differentiation by exposure to lead and cadmium. *Neurotoxicology and Teratology, 14,* 247–252.

Stiles, K., & Bellinger, D. (1993). Neuropsychological correlates of low-level lead exposure in children: A prospective study. *Neurotoxicology and Teratology, 15,* 27–35.

Sullivan, L. (1991). Luncheon remarks. Presented at Preventing Childhood Lead Poisoning. The First Comprehensive National Conference, Washington, DC, October 7, 1991.

Sundstrom, R., Muntzing, K., Kalimo, H., & Sourander, P. (1985). Changes in the integrity of the blood–brain barrier in suckling rats with low dose lead encephalopathy. *Acta Neuropathologica, 68,* 1–9.

Thacker, S., Hoffman, D., Smith, J., Steinberg, K., & Zack, M. (1992). Effect of low-level body burdens of lead on the mental development of children: Limitations of meta-analysis in a review of longitudinal data. *Archives of Environmental Health, 47,* 336–346.

Tiffany-Castiglioni, E., Sierra, E., Wu, J-N., & Rowles, T. (1989). Lead toxicity in neuroglia. *NeuroToxicology, 10,* 417–444.

Tilson, H., Jacobson, J., & Rogan, W. (1990). Polychlorinated biphenyls and the developing nervous system: Cross-species comparisons. *Neurotoxicology and Teratology, 12,* 239–248.

U.S. Environmental Protection Agency. (1986a). *Air Quality Criteria for Lead.* EPA-600/8-83/028aF-dF. Environmental Criteria and Assessment Office, Research Triangle Park, NC 27711.

U.S. Environmental Protection Agency. (1986b). *Reducing Lead in Drinking Water: A Benefit Analysis.* EPA-230-09-86-019. Washington, DC: Office of Policy Planning and Evaluation.

U.S. Environmental Protection Agency. (1990). *Air Quality Criteria for Lead: Supplement to the 1986 Addendum.* EPA-600/08-89/049f. Research Triangle Park, NC, 1990.

Wasserman, G., Graziano, J., Factor-Litvak, P., Popovac, D., Morina, N., Musabegovic, A., Vrenezi, N., Capuni-Paracka, S., Lekic, V., Preteni-Redjepi, E., Hadzialjevic, S., Slavkovich, V., Kline, J., Shrout, P., & Stein, Z. (1992). Independent effects of lead exposure and iron deficiency anemia on developmental outcome at age 2 years. *Journal of Pediatrics, 121,* 695–703.

Weiss, B. (1985). Intersections of psychiatry and toxicology. *International Journal of Mental Health, 14,* 7–25.

Weiss, B. (1988). Quantitative perspectives on behavioral toxicology. *Toxicology Letters, 43,* 285–293.

Wetmur, J., Lehnert, G., & Desnick, R. (1991). The delta-aminolevulinic dehydratase polymorphism: Higher blood lead levels in lead workers and environmentally exposed children with the 1-2 and 2-2 isozymes. *Environmental Research, 56,* 109–119.

Wigg, N., Vimpani, G., McMichael, A., Baghurst, P., Robertson, E., & Roberts, R. (1988). Port Pirie Cohort Study: Childhood blood lead and neuropsychological development at age 2 years. *Journal of Epidemiology and Community Health, 42,* 213–219.

Winneke, G., Kramer, U., Brockhaus, A., Ewers, U., Kujanek, G., Lechner, H., & Janke, W. (1983). Neuropsychological studies in children with elevated tooth-lead concentrations. II. Extended study. *International Archives of Occupational and Environmental Health, 51,* 231–252.

Winneke, G., & Kramer, U. (1984). Neuropsychological effects of lead in children: Interactions with social background variables. *Neuropsychobiology, 11,* 195–202.

Winneke, G., Beginn, U., Ewert, T., Havestadt, C., Kraemer, U., Krause, C., Thron, H., & Wagner, H. (1985). Comparing the effects of perinatal and later childhood lead exposure on neuropsychological outcome. *Environmental Research, 38,* 155–167.

Winneke, G., Brockhaus, A., Collet, W., & Kramer, U. (1989). Modulation of lead-induced performance deficit in children by varying signal rate in a serial choice reaction task. *Neurotoxicology and Teratology, 11,* 587–592.

Winneke, G., Brockhaus, A., Ewers, U., Kramer, U., & Neuf, M. (1990). Results from the European Multicenter study on lead neurotoxicity in children: Implications for risk assessment. *Neurotoxicology and Teratology, 12,* 553–559.

World Health Organization. (in press). *IPCS Environmental Health Criteria for Inorganic Lead.*

Yule, W., Lansdown, R., Millar, I., & Urbanowicz, M-A. (1981). The relationship between blood lead concentrations, intelligence, and attainment in a school population: A pilot study. *Developmental Medicine and Child Neurology, 23,* 567–576.

CHAPTER 3

Advances in Brain Imaging with Children and Adolescents

ERIN D. BIGLER

A few years ago, I speculated on the pressing need for integrating neuroimaging with neuropsychological assessment (Bigler, 1991). That speculation is now reality, partly because of the rapidly improving methods for automated image analysis (see Andreasen, Cizadlo, Harris, Swayze, O'Leary, Cohen, Earhardt, & Yuh, 1993; Robb, 1990; Figure 3.1). Much of this work is based on the obvious premise that if we had a reliable method for quantitatively presenting neuroimaging data, this information should be most helpful in neuropsychologically assessing the patient.

As an introduction to merging neuropsychological assessment with neuroimaging, let us briefly review developments in neuropsychological assessment and neuroimaging that bring these two fields together. To neuropsychological assessment in the last five years we have seen introduced better norms for current tests (more extensive; matched for age, gender, and education) and new tests with standardization practices superior to those for previously used neuropsychologic measures. Accordingly, for many of the neuropsychological tests now in use, the neuropsychologist can compare a patient's performance on a test with others similar in age, educational background, and gender (Heaton, Grant, & Matthews, 1992). This type of comparative analysis helps immensely in looking at the effects of a lesion or neurologic state because the patient's performance can be compared directly to the norm reference group and deviations will stand out. Much neuropsychological work in the past has dealt with "cut-off scores" or some type of binary classification of patients (i.e., organic vs. nonorganic—the patient either meets criteria for "brain damage" or does not). We can now much better appreciate the continuum of effects of brain injury on neuropsychological performance and neurologic states rather than settle for a kind of binary classification. This improvement applies particularly to children because of the requirement that we always consider developmental features.

Neuroimaging exhibits a similar trend. Historically, radiology, at one level, was as much an art as it was a science (Eisenberg, 1992); the field of radiology often looked at pathology as a binary classification as well

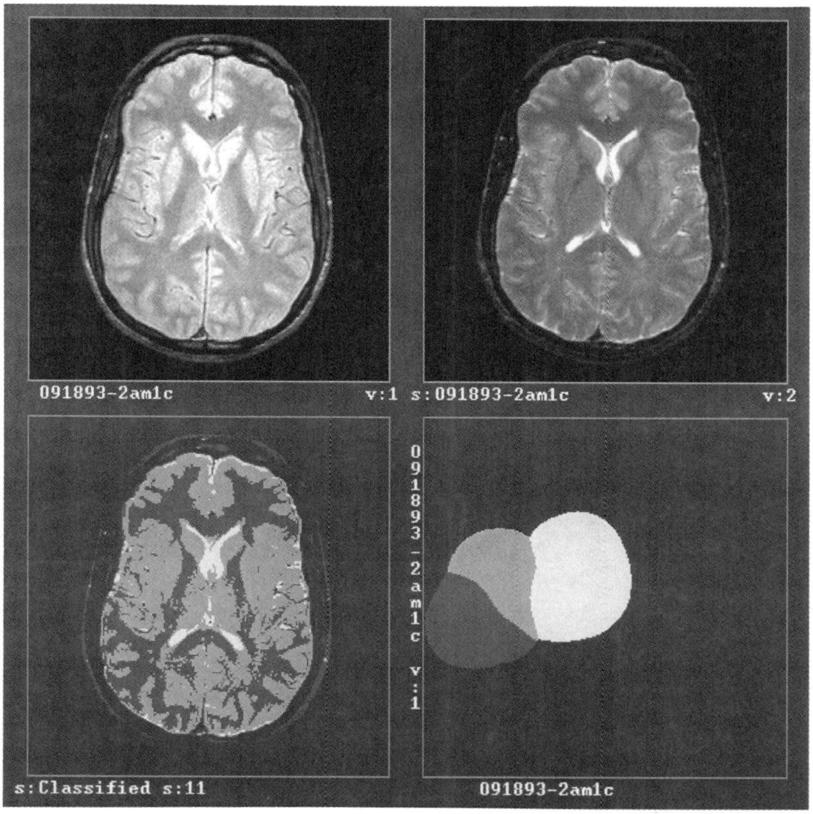

Fig. 3.1. Multispectral segmentation of MR images. Upper left: intermediate, and (upper right) T_2-weighted spin-echo images at the level of the body of the lateral ventricles. Operator-identified regions of interest for CSF at lower left, where light gray represents CSF, intermediate gray represents gray matter, and white matter as dark gray. Lower right: Plot of two-dimensional feature space, where each pixel is plotted with the signal intensity on the T_2-weighted image as the x-axis and the signal intensity on the intermediate-weighted image as the y-axis. The location in feature space of the pixels obtained in the user-identified regions are shown in their respective colors. Lower left: 2-D feature space after applying the k-nearest-neighbor segmentation algorithm demonstrating the feature space regions assigned to each segmented tissue type. These techniques, pioneered by Robb, allow for automated image analysis to quantify almost any anatomic structure. (Figure produced using ANALYZE^{TM}, Biomedical Imaging Resource, Mayo Foundation.)

(i.e., abnormal vs. normal). The radiologic interpretation was based on what the radiologist "saw" and, in that sense, interpretation was in the eye of the beholder. In the past, as depicted in Figure 3.2, a radiologic report of a child with hydrocephalus typically made statements such as "enlarged ventricular system" but provided no quantification for the

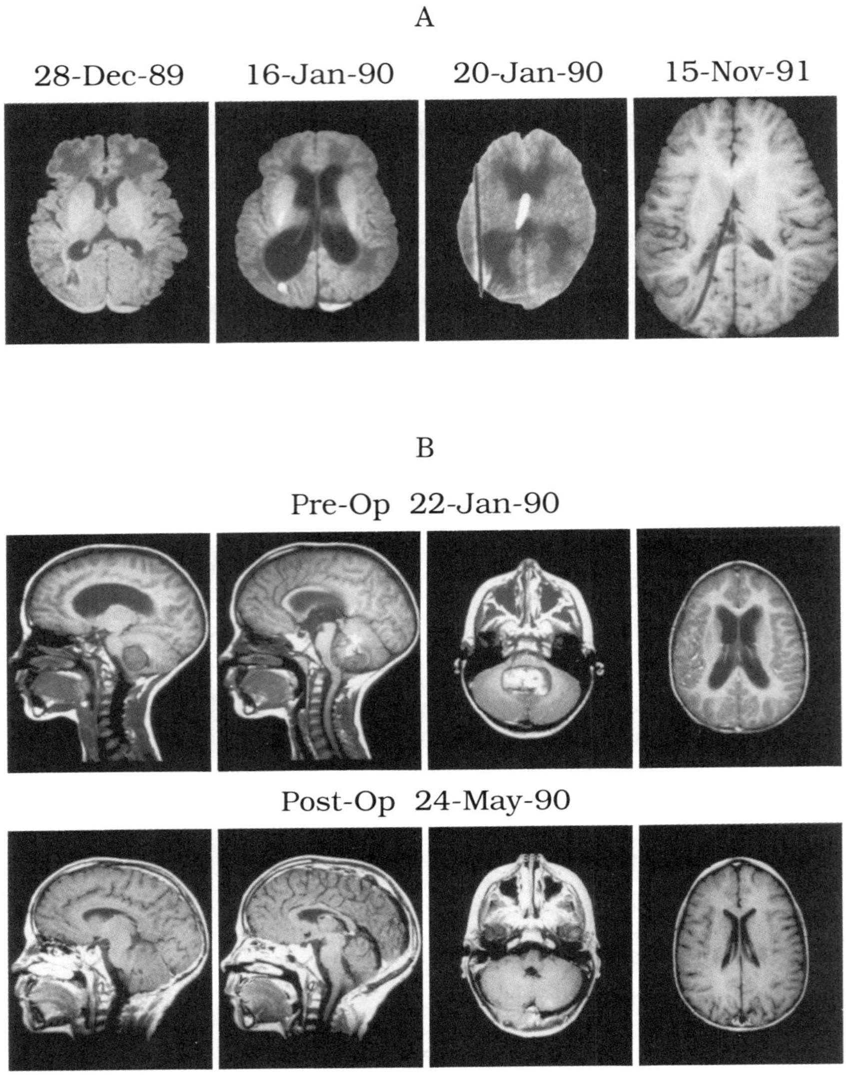

Fig. 3.2. (A) Sequential views of progressive hydrocephalus followed by ventricular reduction post-shunting. These imaging studies clearly demonstrate the enlargement of the ventricular system and pathologic changes that have occurred in this child's brain. The tradition in neuroradiology, however, has been not to quantify these changes. Thus, one can look at this study and visually inspect the record and clearly see the changes (particularly from December 28 to January 16), but in the past these changes have typically been reported without quantification. (B) Sequential views pre- and postsurgery in a child with cerebellar tumor. Same comments as above. Past visualizations generally did not quantify the size of the tumor and the effects on surrounding tissue as well as degree of nonspecific effect (volume of hydrocephalic development). The future of the neuroradiology–neuropsychology interface is in quantifying these changes and determining how these quantifications relate to systematic changes in behavior and function.

degree of ventricular enlargement and potential degradation or degeneration of cortical and subcortical structures. Likewise, the report of a post-tumor resection magnetic resonance scan of a child in the past might have mentioned of "post-craniectomy findings and surgical removal with encephalomalacic changes surrounding the original lesion site, otherwise within normal limits" (see Figure 3.2b also), but provided no quantification of pathologic change. Currently, all these qualitative statements can be bolstered with quantitative measurements of the brain and pathologic changes that may be present.

In this chapter we review contemporary quantitative neuroimaging methods and conclude with various ways of displaying neuroimaging data and how these data can be related to neuropsychological assessment.

Quantitative Neuroimaging

With quantitative neuroimaging, any target brain structure can be made a region of interest (ROI), as illustrated in Figure 3.3. In this figure, the ventricle and corpus callosum are the target structures or ROIs and their outer boundary is traced. This delineation in turn permits us to quantify a surface area at that level of the brain. By identifying the position of each slice and the distance between slices that contain the ROI, surface areas can be turned into structure volume. Because of variability in head size, some correction factor is needed and two methods are presented in Figure 3.3. With this technology, a normative database can be developed for various anatomic structures. Table 3.1 provides data on the lateral ventricular system and corpus callosum for ages 16 to 65 (see Blatter, Bigler, Gale, Johnson, Anderson, Burnett, Kurth, & Horn, in press).

With Table 3.1, the clinician or researcher can approach the problem of ascertaining the degree of deviation in findings on corpus callosum and ventricular volume in a subject by comparing the subject's measured value to the table. In Figure 3.4, three TBI cases are compared to a normal subject and to the normative data on corpus callosum morphology.

We and others have sought to expand this approach to include multiple cortical and subcortical measures (see Blatter et al., in press; Pfefferbaum Mathalon, Sullivan, Rawles, Zipursky, & Lim, in press). This information is presented in Table 3.2, displaying the quantity of whole-brain cerebral spinal fluid, subarachnoid cerebral spinal fluid, various ventricular measurements, along with white and gray matter, and a ventricle-to-brain ratio. This information can be used as a working database for comparing deviation in any structure in any individual.

With these approaches in mind, a case study can be usefully illustrative, as in Figure 3.5. This patient sustained a significant TBI in a fall while mountain climbing. He sustained a basilar skull fracture and bifrontal contusions with a large hemorrhagic contusion and subdural hematoma in

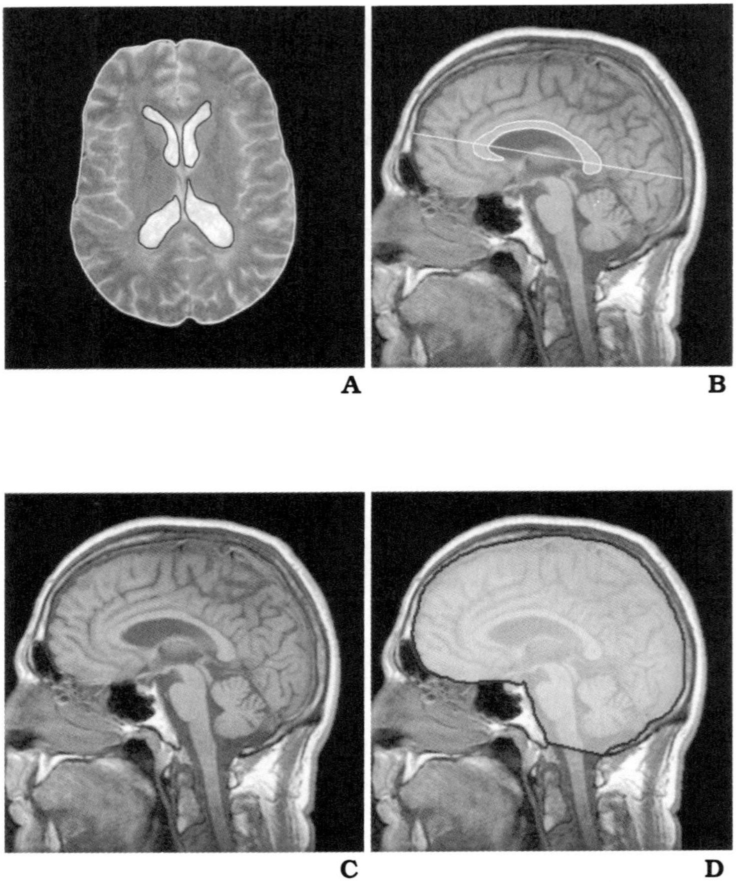

Fig. 3.3. Methods of quantification: (a) Axial view with the outer rim of the anterior horns and atrial/posterior horns of the lateral ventricle. This view permits calculation of the surface area of the ventricular system at that level. By taking each slice wherein the ventricle is present along with the known distance between slices, a structure volume can be calculated. In this illustration, the outer rim of the brain is traced in white. This calculation can be used as a correction factor at this level to control for head size. Similarly, by taking each slice, total brain volume can be estimated. (b) Saggital view, mesial surface area of the brain with the corpus callosum outlined in white. This outline can also be used to quantify the mesial surface area of the corpus callosum. The linear anterior-to-posterior line provides a direct measure of internal skull length, which also can be used as a correction factor for head size. (c and d) Saggital view of the mesial surface of the brain, with intracranial content outlined in (d). This view also provides a measure of intracranial size. The base of the outline is at the level of the foramen magnum.

Table 3.1.A. Corpus callosum average area across gender and age.

Females Age	*n*	CC (mm^2)	SD	cc/miss	SD
16–25	20	675	112	4.2	0.598
26–35	21	650	67	4.24	0.418
36–45	20	692	81	4.3	0.411
46–55	22	652	107	4.14	0.49
56–65	14	629	93	4.12	0.614
Totals	$n = 97$	avg = 661	94	4.20	0.499

Males Age	*n*	CC (mm^2)	SD	cc/miss	SD
16–25	28	690	88	4.05	0.504
26–35	21	685	79	4.05	0.452
36–45	13	687	106	4.12	0.570
46–55	17	685	87	4.25	0.404
56–65	13	632	78	3.78	0.400
Totals	$n = 92$	avg = 680	87	4.06	0.480

Table 3.1.B. Normative quantitative neuroimaging data by decade and gender for 189 normal and medical control individuals.

Uncorrected females	Total ventricle mean	SD	Lateral ventricle mean	SD	L temp horn mean	SD	R temp horn mean	VBR[a] mean	SD
16–25	17.25	4.95	14.44	4.65	0.19	0.09	0.20	1.31	0.35
26–35	16.83	7.49	14.31	7.14	0.17	0.17	0.23	1.36	0.59
36–45	15.18	4.44	12.58	4.14	0.21	0.24	0.17	1.22	0.33
46–55	15.95	4.45	13.43	4.34	0.13	0.07	0.18	1.23	0.29
56–65	20.70	9.53	17.73	8.86	0.18	0.24	0.25	1.72	0.81
Males									
16–25	17.85	6.27	15.06	6.01	0.16	0.11	0.19	1.21	0.42
26–35	20.08	7.11	16.66	6.95	0.18	0.15	0.26	1.38	0.42
36–45	18.99	5.95	15.33	5.74	0.24	0.20	0.23	1.35	0.44
46–55	20.98	5.39	17.98	5.17	0.16	0.14	0.18	1.51	0.42
56–65	34.74	13.57	31.19	13.08	0.26	0.23	0.30	2.50	0.92

Corrected females	Total ventricle mean	SD	Lateral ventricle mean	SD	L temp horn mean	SD	R temp horn mean	VBR[a] mean	SD
16–25	1.23%	4.97	1.03%	4.66	0.014%	0.09	0.014%	1.23%	0.35
26–35	1.26%	7.68	1.07%	7.33	0.013%	0.17	0.017%	1.26%	0.61
36–45	1.12%	4.58	0.93%	4.31	0.015%	0.25	0.013%	1.12%	0.34
46–55	1.13%	4.85	0.95%	4.81	0.009%	0.07	0.013%	1.13%	0.33
56–65	1.53%	9.41	1.31%	8.75	0.013%	0.24	0.018%	1.53%	0.80
Males									
16–25	1.14%	5.94	0.96%	5.76	0.010%	0.11	0.012%	1.14%	0.40
26–35	1.29%	7.58	1.07%	7.34	0.012%	0.15	0.017%	1.29%	0.45
36–45	1.22%	6.10	0.99%	5.86	0.015%	0.20	0.015%	1.22%	0.45
46–55	1.36%	5.89	1.17%	5.65	0.010%	0.14	0.012%	1.36%	0.47
56–65	2.19%	7.42	1.96%	7.59	0.016%	0.20	0.019%	2.19%	0.50

[a] Based in part on material from Blatter et al., 1994.

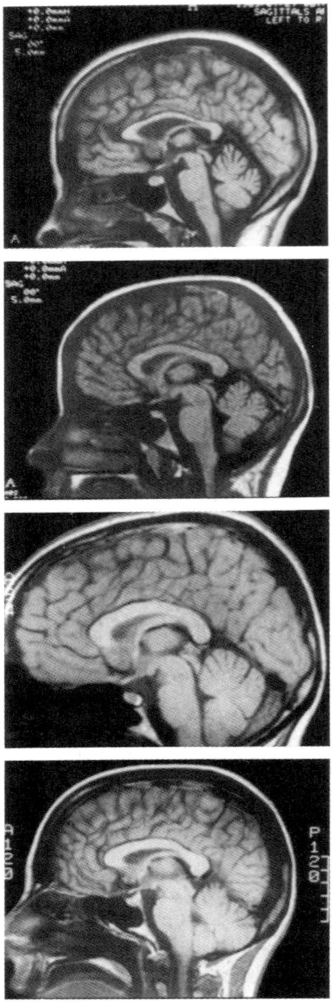

Area 449.63mm^2
VBR 3.1

Area 557.07mm^2
M ± SD569.9mm^2 ± 15.2mm^2
VBR 2.37± 1.37

Area 740.38mm^2
M ± SD684.6mm^2 ± 73.1mm^2
VBR 2.83 ± 1.51

Area 699.42mm^2
M ± SD696.9mm^2 ± 44.8mm^2
VBR 1.40 ± 0.55

Fig. 3.4. The top three scans are from patients with traumatic brain injury of varying severity (top: severe; second from top: moderate; second from bottom: mild; bottom: normal control). The bottom scan is a midsaggital view from a normal subject, depicting normal size and morphology of the corpus callosum.

the right frontal area that was surgically evacuated. The magnetic resonance studies were done approximately two years postinjury and demonstrate significant changes, particularly in the frontal region of the brain (see Figure 3.5). Comparing aspects of this patient's morphometric data to the normal database demonstrates a significant change in the size of the ventricular system with significant wasting of the frontal area. These findings can then be compared with the neuropsychological data presented

Table 3.2. Normative quantitative neuroimaging data by decade and gender for 189 normal and medical control individuals.

Uncorrected females	n	Age mean	SD	Total CSF[a] mean	SD	Subarachnoid CSF mean	SD	SD	III mean	SD	IV mean	SD	GM mean	SD	WM mean	SD	Total brain mean	SD
16–25	16	20.44	3.0	83.36	34.23	66.11	30.27	0.10	0.68	0.18	1.73	0.55	709.18	109.43	605.16	104.27	1,314.35	71.81
26–35	23	30.83	3.2	92.85	37.13	76.02	33.59	0.33	0.65	0.26	1.47	0.41	648.27	105.28	590.78	86.76	1,239.06	103.22
36–45	20	40.00	2.8	110.43	32.57	95.25	30.76	0.14	0.66	0.29	1.55	0.34	621.88	107.57	623.47	113.52	1,245.35	111.70
46–55	15	50.40	2.6	117.95	28.27	102.00	27.24	0.12	0.73	0.25	1.48	0.47	581.54	108.17	709.96	92.05	1,291.49	129.77
56–65	13	59.54	2.0	140.06	31.13	119.36	30.14	0.22	0.96	0.36	1.57	0.42	611.72	81.64	602.50	110.52	1,214.23	115.43
Males																		
16–25	22	22.90	2.0	89.82	31.93	71.97	30.03	0.11	0.70	0.22	1.74	0.58	757.48	106.85	719.42	98.24	1,476.90	114.56
26–35	17	31.47	3.1	121.93	32.96	101.84	30.53	0.16	0.79	0.24	2.19	0.58	780.52	79.08	660.19	96.77	1,440.71	97.45
36–45	13	41.31	2.8	140.07	42.68	121.08	40.15	0.21	1.08	0.40	2.11	0.56	724.24	104.80	689.01	119.00	1,413.25	85.24
46–55	16	50.88	2.5	141.54	38.84	102.56	37.90	0.10	1.13	0.38	1.53	0.52	719.53	65.76	678.25	121.42	1,397.77	143.74
56–65	11	62.09	4.0	206.20	72.82	171.45	70.00	0.21	1.49	0.76	1.51	0.23	709.04	173.94	674.69	148.32	1,383.72	133.27

Corrected females	n	Age mean	SD	Total CSF[a] mean	SD	Subarachnoid CSF mean	SD	SD	III mean	SD	IV mean	SD	GM mean	SD	WM mean	SD	Total brain mean	SD
16–25	14	20.43	3.2	5.96%	36.13	4.73%	31.94	0.10	0.05%	0.18	0.13%	0.56	51.37%	107.81	43.84%	108.53	94.04%	74.72
26–35	21	30.90	3.1	6.97%	36.68	5.71%	32.83	0.34	0.05%	0.25	0.11%	0.41	49.30%	109.72	44.92%	90.58	93.03%	108.16
36–45	18	40.00	2.9	8.15%	28.49	7.03%	26.80	0.14	0.05%	0.19	0.12%	0.35	46.39%	98.48	46.51%	108.34	91.85%	117.83
46–55	9	49.60	2.8	8.37%	29.95	7.24%	29.05	0.13	0.05%	0.25	0.11%	0.51	41.73%	115.06	50.95%	85.80	91.63%	89.62
56–65	14	59.30	2.1	10.34%	31.77	8.81%	30.21	0.21	0.07%	0.35	0.12%	0.40	45.87%	84.04	45.18%	110.43	89.66%	110.91
Males																		
16–25	21	22.90	2.1	5.73%	32.62	4.59%	30.77	0.11	0.05%	0.22	0.11%	0.55	48.91%	104.53	46.45%	100.13	94.27%	109.24
26–35	16	31.60	3.2	7.80%	37.99	6.52%	34.88	0.16	0.05%	0.24	0.14%	0.56	50.60%	78.75	42.80%	92.13	92.20%	99.05
36–45	11	41.60	2.9	9.02%	42.10	7.79%	40.11	0.22	0.07%	0.41	0.14%	0.60	47.20%	100.68	44.91%	118.08	90.98%	89.98
46–55	13	50.40	2.5	9.20%	35.45	6.66%	34.09	0.10	0.08%	0.41	0.10%	0.53	47.96%	62.47	45.21%	134.21	90.80%	154.10
56–65	8	62.10	3.5	12.97%	75.60	10.78%	77.30	0.16	0.10%	0.85	0.10%	0.25	45.59%	163.94	43.38%	132.93	87.03%	147.86

[a] Based in part on material from Blatter et al., 1994.

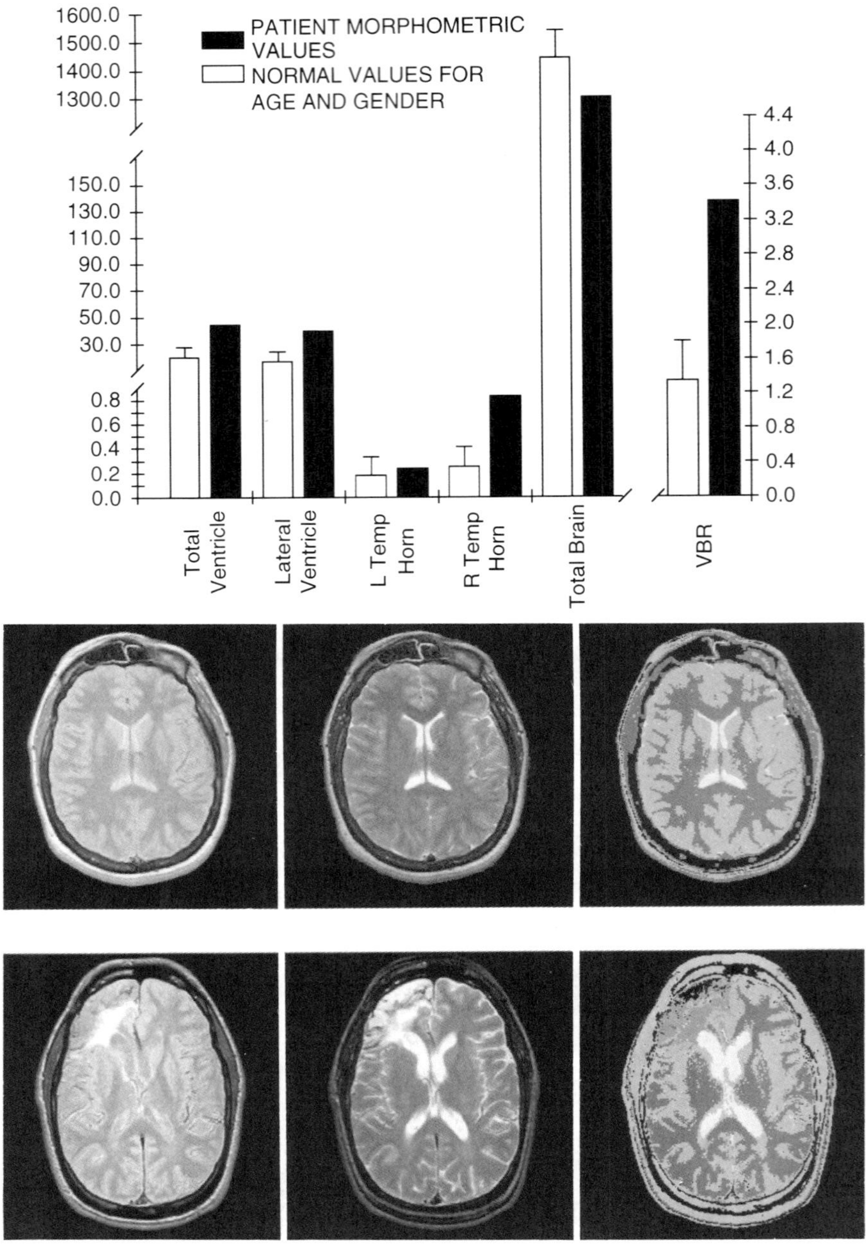

Fig. 3.5. Bar graph depicting aspects of the patient's quantitative neuroimaging findings about the ventricular system, based on volumetric estimates from segmented images. See Table 3.1 for the complete array of neuroimaging data on the ventricular system. The top row of MR images depict a medical control subject with proton density-weighted MR scan on the left, T_2-weighted scan in the middle, and the "segmented" image differentiating white, gray, and CSF space. The bottom row of images is from the TBI patient with MR images at a similar level and a large right frontal lesion (left is at the reader's right). The patient's neuropsychological data are presented in Table 3.4. These quantitative analyses indicate significant ventricular dilation, which, in TBI, is a sign of white-matter loss. (Adapted by Bigler, 1990.)

in Figure 3.6. We fully discuss how this information can be utilized in the legends accompanying Figures 3.4 and 3.5.

This movement toward quantifying neuroanatomic abnormalities is added to the continued emphasis on clinical descriptors of imaging abnormalities in various neurologic disorders (see Barkovich, 1990; Barkovich, Chuang, & Norman, 1988; Barkovich & Kjos, 1992a; Barkovich & Kjos, 1992b; Barkovich & Norman, 1989; Kjos, Umansky, & Barkovich, 1990; Wolpert & Barnes, 1992). Because MR imaging is a relatively new procedure, we still need thorough qualitative description of the type of abnormalities seen in various neurologic disorders. As indicated above, though, merely describing these abnormalities is no longer sufficient: the abnormalities should also be quantified. We anticipate that this quantification will lead to even better clinical description of the abnormalities present in imaging in children with neurologic disorder.

Presenting Three-Dimensional Imaging

The quest in neuroimaging has been methods for visualizing cerebral structures in the best possible fashion. Neuroimaging history is based on technological advances that provide enhanced in vivo visualization of the target anatomic structure (Oldendorf, 1980). Until recently, these methods have been relegated to two-dimensional, single-plane views based on CT, MR, or related imaging technology (Eisenberg, 1992). With recent advances in technology, however, excellent 3-D reconstruction can now be achieved in both CT and MR platforms, which can be used to superimpose Positron Emission Tomography (PET) and Single Photon Emission Computed Tomography (SPECT), which have less resolving power.

The predecessor of 3-D imaging was the ability of MR imaging to represent the brain in sections and planes (see Figure 3.7). This type of data analysis now enables us to produce contemporary 3-D brain images, as presented in Figure 3.8. This method, in turn, permits 3-D reconstruction of any brain-surface area in any orientation desired. As in this figure, 3-D representation of the whole brain is excellent. This method provides an effective means for depicting cortical abnormalities, but "see-through" techniques are probably best for visualizing and quantifying subcortical areas, as discussed below.

Along these lines, we have devised techniques using a wire-frame outline of the brain and the ventricle as the base structure. The ventricle is included for a straightforward reason (Bigler, 1992a): Ventricular expansion is a sign of parenchymal tissue degeneration and the direction of change within the ventricular system relates to the region of greatest parenchymal degeneration. For example, in TBI, if the frontal area of the brain is most damaged, one typically sees more dilation of the anterior horns than of any other aspect of the lateral ventricular system, as

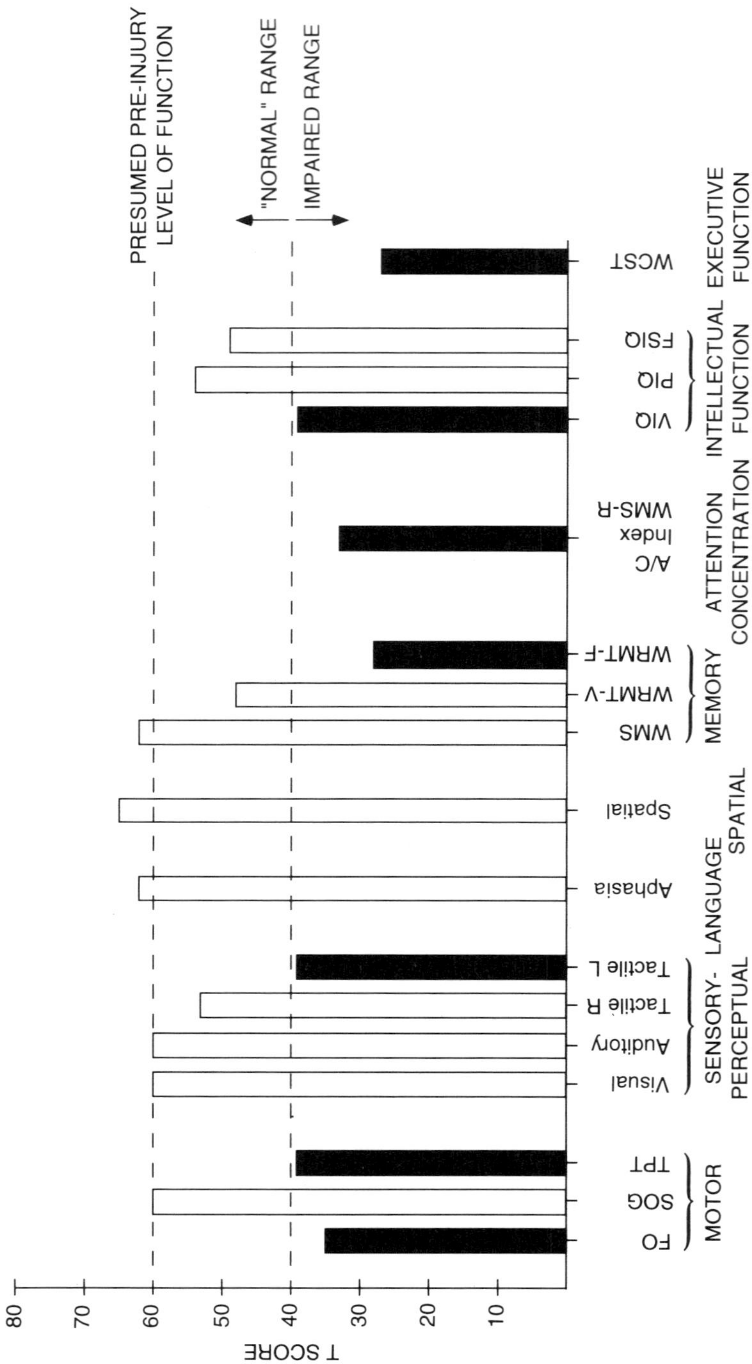

PRESUMED PRE-INJURY LEVEL OF FUNCTION
"NORMAL" RANGE
IMPAIRED RANGE
T SCORE
80
70
60
50
40
30
20
10
FO
SOG
TPT
MOTOR
Visual
Auditory
Tactile R
Tactile L
SENSORY-PERCEPTUAL
Aphasia
LANGUAGE
Spatial
SPATIAL
WMS
WRMT-V
WRMT-F
MEMORY
A/C Index WMS-R
ATTENTION CONCENTRATION
VIQ
PIQ
FSIQ
INTELLECTUAL FUNCTION
WCST
EXECUTIVE FUNCTION

depicted in Figure 3.9. Also, in traumatic brain injury, there is often a generalized increase in overall ventricular size because of the relationship between white-matter injury effects and ventricular dilation (see Bigler, 1992b). Much of the periventricular space is surrounded by white matter, in particular the corpus callosum (see Figure 3.10). Accordingly, in cases of TBI, the white matter degenerates, which, in turn, results in passive expansion of the ventricular system. This result is demonstrated in Figure 3.11, wherein the day-of-injury CT scan is used to determine an estimate

←

Fig. 3.6. Neuropsychological performance of the patient depicted in Fig. 3.4. The x-axis lists neuropsychological test findings with the scores converted into a T-score for direct comparison (mean = 50, standard deviation = 10) along the y-axis. Abbreviations: FO = finger oscillation; SOG = strength of grip; TPT = Tactual Performance Test; AST = Aphasia Screening Test; WMS-R = Wechsler Memory Scale-Revised; WRMT-V = Warrington Recognition Memory Test-Verbal; WRMT-F = Warrington Recognition Memory Test-Faces; A/C Index = Attention/Concentration Index; VIQ = Verbal Intellectual Quotient; PIQ = Performance Intellectual Quotient; FSIQ = Full Scale Intellectual Quotient based on the results of the Wechsler Adult Intelligence Scale-Revised (1981); WCST = Wisconsin Card Sorting Test. This neuropsychological profile indicates that the patient has no deficit in basic motor strength, as reflected by the intact SOG scores. Fine motor movement (FO), however, as well as integrative motor control (TPT) is below what would be expected to be normal. Sensory-perceptual examination reveals intact visual and auditory processing, bilaterally, but the patient has diminished tactile perceptual processing on the left compared to the right. No deficits are seen in Language, Spatial, and General Memory Index score on the Wechsler Memory Scale-Revised. Clearly, however, he has a deficit in facial recognition memory on the Warrington Recognition Memory Test compared to a normal WMS-R General Memory Index and a normal performance on the Warrington Recognition Memory Test for Words (Verbal). The patient's Attention/Concentration Index was distinctly impaired on the WMS-R. His intellectual functioning is probably below what would be predicted given his premorbid ability level. He has a distinct deficit in ability to perform the Wisconsin Card Sort task, which places demands on flexible thinking and cognitive shifting, typically deficit areas for patients with significant frontal-lobe damage. This patient was a very successful contractor and builder who sustained a serious traumatic brain injury in a 70-foot fall while rock climbing. He had graduated from high school and had completed four years of college but had not graduated. Both parents were college educated and his father was a university professor. Accordingly, this patient's preinjury intellectual/cognitive status was felt to be in the above-average range, as depicted by the horizontal line. Taken together, these neuropsychological findings suggest a defect in frontal-lobe function, with lateralization to the right hemisphere. Accordingly, these neuropsychological findings are consistent with the neuroimaging findings presented in the MR scans in Fig. 3.4.

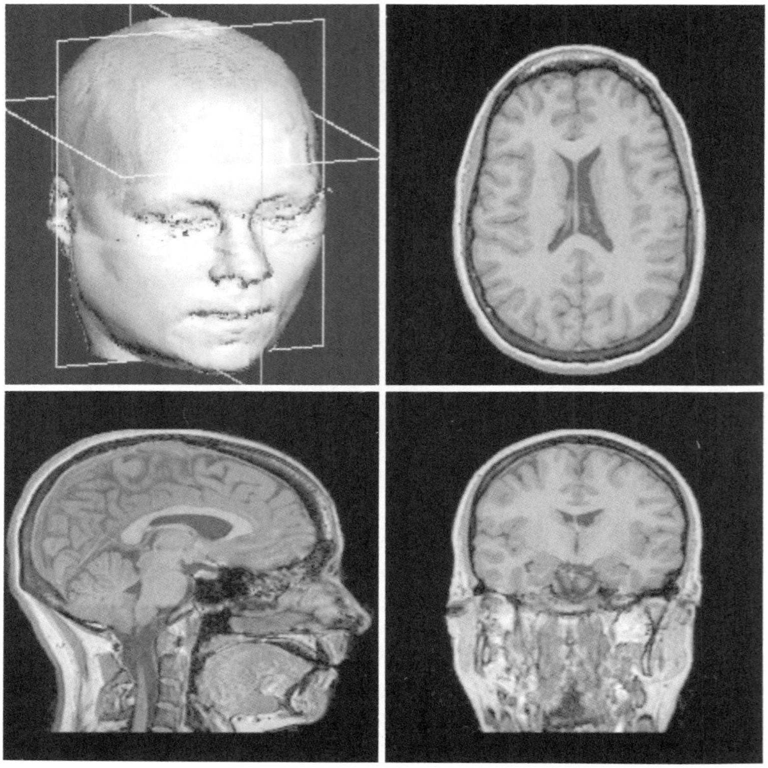

Fig. 3.7. A traditional 2-D depiction of multiple MR slices taken at various brain-section levels with a 3-D MR-based depiction of the head demonstrating the three planes of anatomic sectioning. (Reprinted with permission by, Richard A. Robb, Mayo Foundation/Clinic, Rochester, MN based on The ANALYZE image analysis program.)

of preinjury morphology. Marked changes in ventricular size are readily documented with these techniques.

Similar techniques work well in depicting pathologic changes in children with a variety of conditions. In Figures 3.11, 3.12, and 3.13, the CT scan prepared closest to the time of birth provides a baseline from which to document significant pathological changes.

Integration

The approach that is on the horizon is integrating quantitative neuropsychological assessment with quantitative neuroimaging. Turkheimer and his colleagues (Turkheimer, 1989; Turkheimer, Cullum, Hubler,

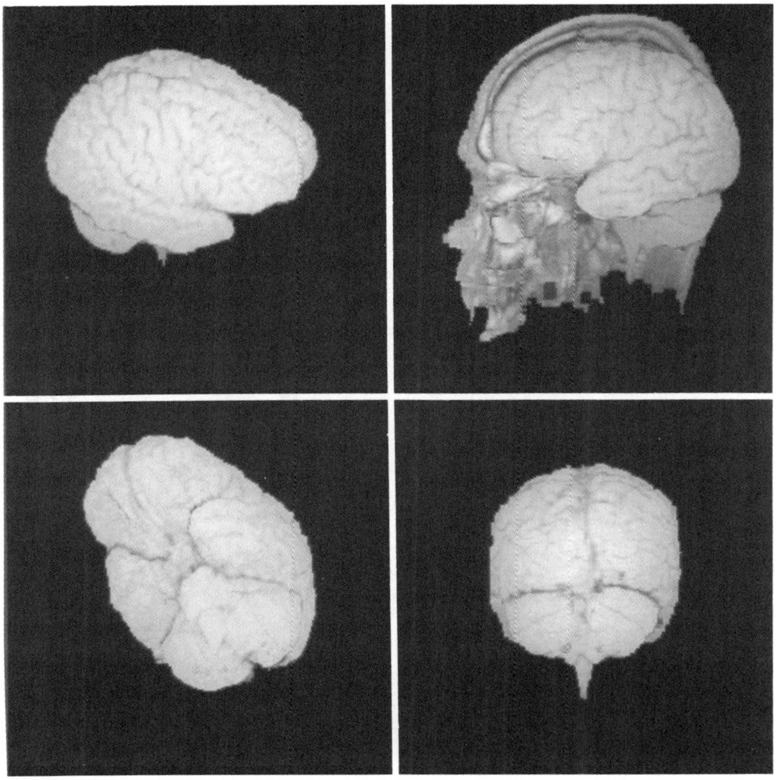

Fig. 3.8. 3-D surface rendering of the human brain based on MR imaging. The top-right view shows the brain in situ. The other three images are with the brain segmented away from bone and meninges. Top left: Lateral view of right hemisphere. Bottom left: Inferior oblique. Right bottom: Posterior.

Paver, Yeo, & Bigler, 1984; Turkheimer, Yeo, Jones, & Bigler, 1990; Turkheimer, Yeo, Jones, & Bigler, 1990) suggest using importance functions to integrate neuroimaging and neuropsychological findings. This subject is thoroughly discussed in previous publications (see Bigler, 1991). Because the importance function was based on the premise of two-dimensionality, the current direction of this research obviously has to involve three-dimensional representation of the brain. At this time, several options are being explored. The outcome is likely to be a way of visualizing the data in one scan image with a type of rating system superimposed upon the lesion and nonlesioned regions of the brain. Until agreement is reached on how to display these findings, the traditional approach of showing some type of comparative, two-dimensional view will probably remain with use.

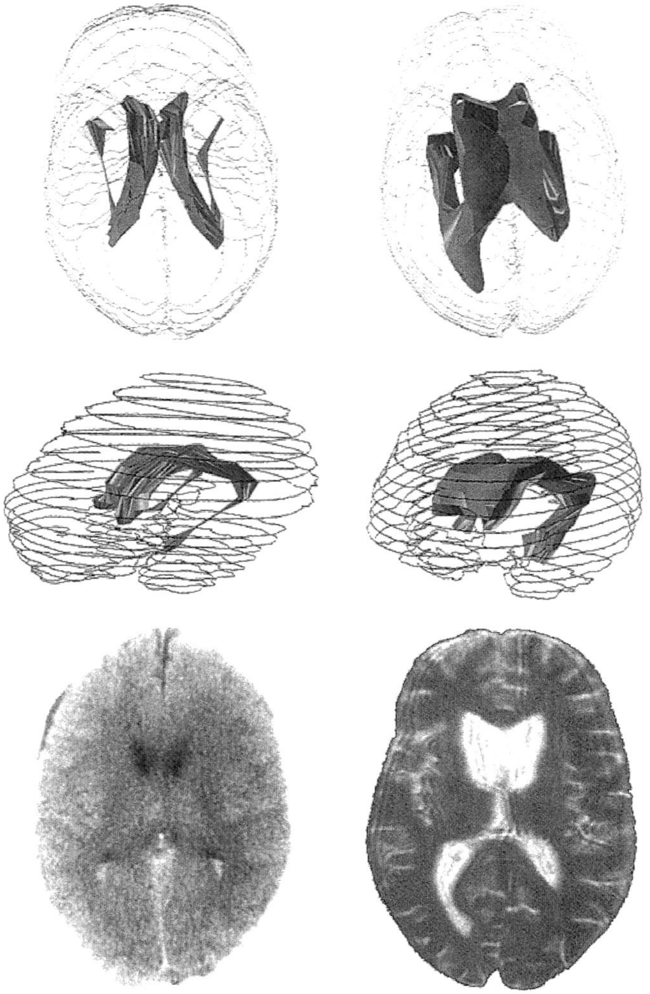

Fig. 3.9. Left: Day-of-injury CT scan and 3-dimensional rendering of the ventricular system. Right: MR imaging depicting marked ventricular dilation, which is represented in the 3-D imaging above the MR scan. This case demonstrates the utility of using day-of-injury information to compare postinjury degenerative changes. As can be seen, differences are clear, particularly in size and configuration of inferior and anterior horn of the lateral ventricular system. This difference indicates frontal- and temporal-lobe pathologic changes, typical changes observed in TBI. (Adapted by Bigler, 1990.)

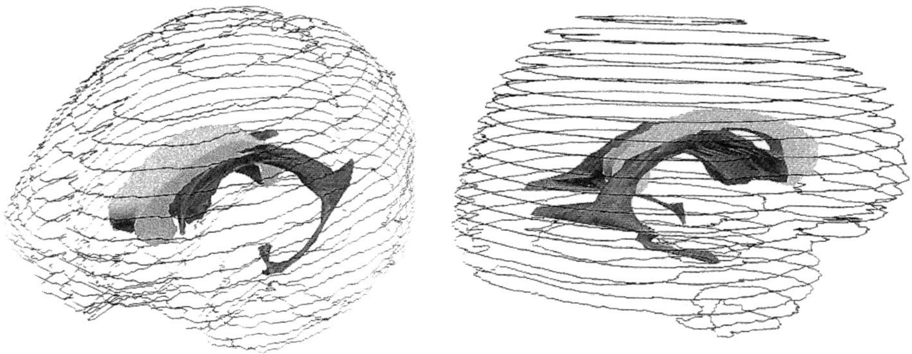

Fig. 3.10. Three-dimensional wire-frame depiction of the corpus callosum in relation to the ventricular system. The point in this illustration is how the corpus callosum wraps around the lateral ventricles. Accordingly, a change in white-matter status that results in degradation of the corpus callosum will result in ventricular dilation. Hence, the ventricle can be used as a "window" into brain morphology.

Several interesting comparative studies have been done. Reiss and colleagues (1993a,b) have studied volumetric changes in Rett Syndrome, a disorder that results in mental retardation and a host of severe neurologic problems, as well as volumetric differences in monozygotic twins discordant for Turner's Syndrome. Their findings are presented in Figures 3.14 and 3.15, and Tables 3.3, 3.4, and 3.5. Here, the authors present two-dimensional comparisons at equally registered anatomic sites based on MR imaging. In both of these studies, direct comparison to normal, matched controls allows immediate visualization of pathologic changes or differences in the presenting neurologic condition. The neuropsychological data in Tables 3.3–3.5 directly compare pathologic conditions and normal controls for neuropsychological performance (comparing each domain). In the future neuroimaging and neuropsychology will have this type of direct side-by-side data comparison for immediate visual inspection of both the imaging data and the neuropsychological performance.

Finally, the quantitative neuroimaging approach has potential for diagnostically classifying clinical groups. For example, a significant amount of research has been focused on imaging in children with developmental and learning disorders (see Bigler, 1992a; Jernigan, Hesselink, Sowell, & Tallal, 1991; Leonard, Voeller, Lombardino, Morris, Hynd, Alexander, Andersen, Garofalakis, Honeyman, Mao, Agge, & Staab, 1993). Although recent work by Schultz et al. (in press) has not found significant volume changes in the left temporal and perisylvian regions of the brain as others have, some type of biological marker may be present in the

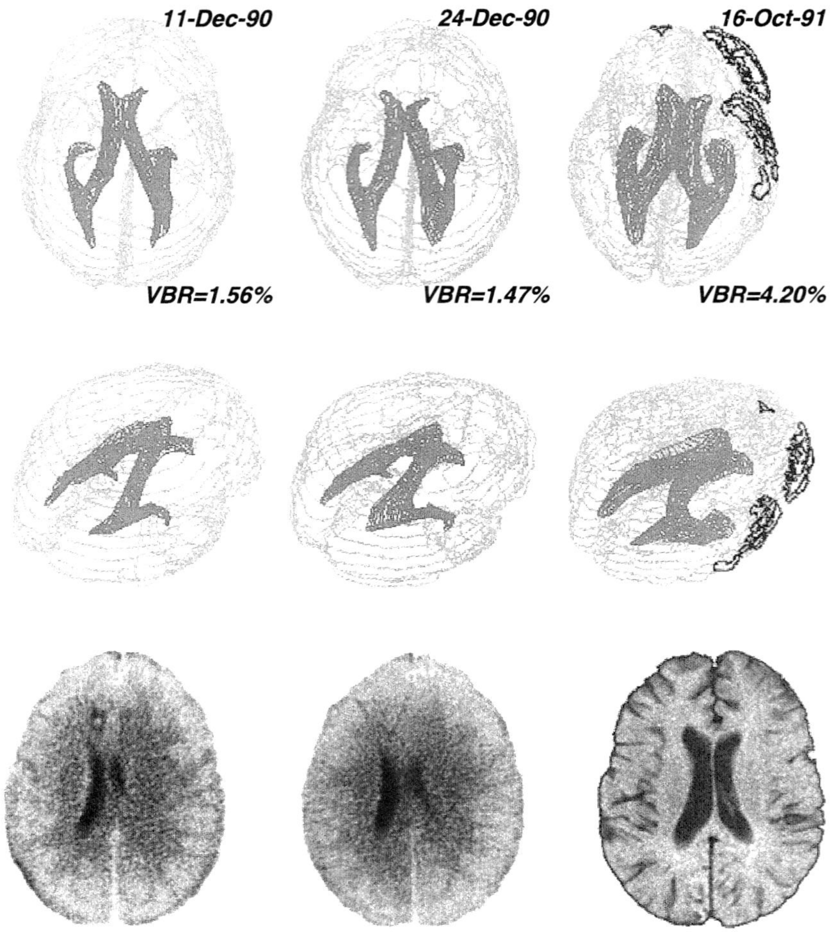

Fig. 3.11(A). Top left: Three-dimensional dorsal view of the ventricular system on the day of injury. Middle: Two weeks later. Top right: 10 months postinjury. The VBR is presented below The top image for each separate analysis performed. A normal VBR is typically in the range of 1.50, indicating that the acute VBR in these patients is in the normal range, but it changes dramatically with the onset of degenerative effects of postinjury. The corresponding neuroimaging data are presented below.

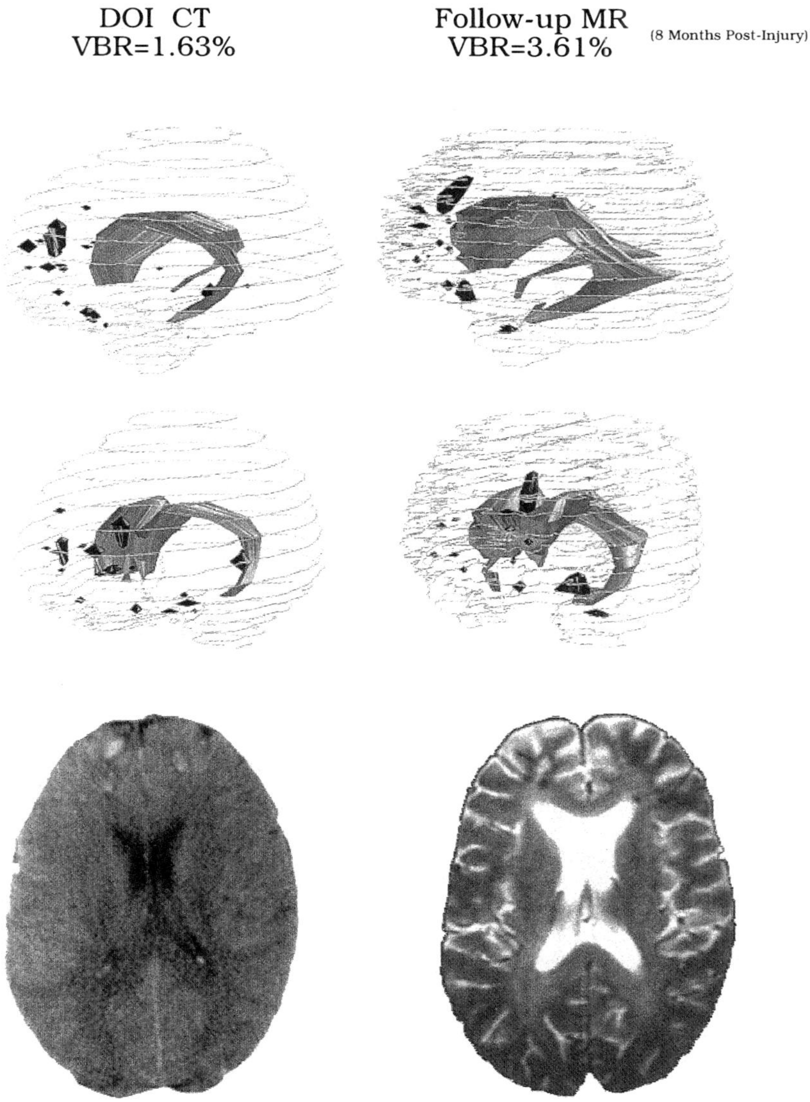

Fig. 3.11(B). Left column: 3-D image representation of the ventricular system and location of cortical and subcortical hemorrhagic contusions. Day-of-injury CT scan is depicted at bottom left. Right: A right-column-match 3-D depiction and representation of the ventricular system two years postinjury, with MR scan at bottom depicting ventricular dilation and presence of necrotic lesions secondary to the subcortical hemorrhagic foci. These lesions are represented in white and off shades of gray as well, although they are not acute lesions, as in the left-hand column.

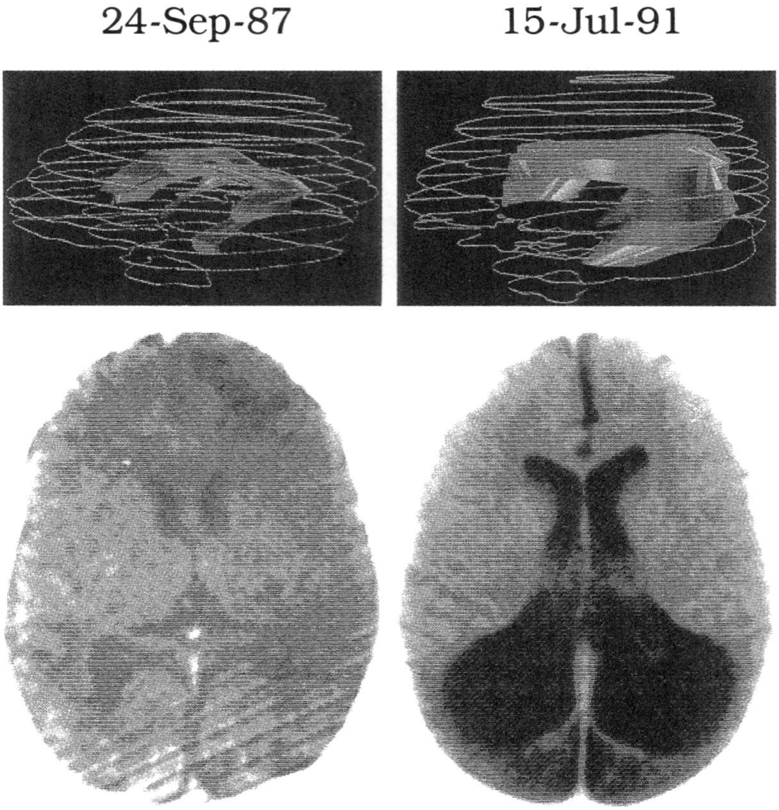

Fig. 3.12. Left-hand column: 3-dimensional ventricular representation on early CT scan done several days postbirth following a complicated delivery. Notice the size and configuration of the ventricular system early in this infant's life. Right-hand column: Significant ventricular enlargement along with major structural changes in the posterior aspect of this child's brain are demonstrated in the follow-up CT and 3-dimensional representation.

child with learning disorder that might lend itself to earlier detection. Throughout the remainder of this decade, research in neuroimaging and neuropsychological diagnostics will be focused on trying to identify such biologic and neuropsychological markers to help diagnose and classify neurologic disease states. These issues are discussed further in the next section.

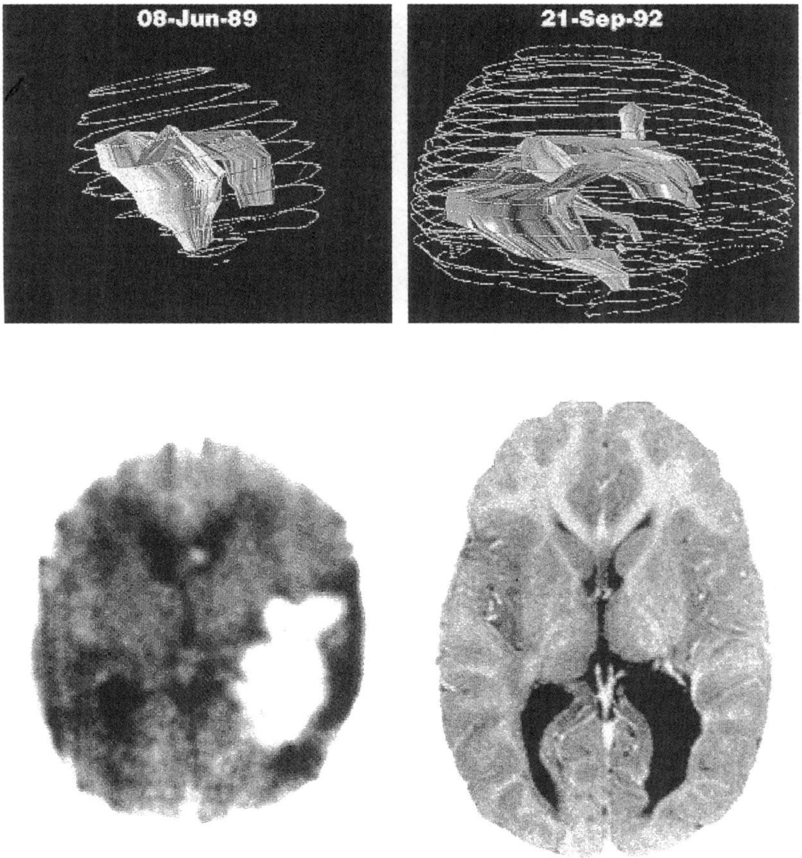

Fig. 3.13. Left-hand column: Traumatic hemorrhage related to a complicated birth and delivery. The hemorrhage is quite massive and in the posterior right hemisphere. Right-hand column: 3-dimensional image reconstruction showing the position and location of ventricular changes secondary to the original hemorrhagic lesion effect.

New Imaging Methods

A variety of new imaging methods that hold promise in pediatric neuroimaging will, in turn, be relevant for pediatric neuropsychology. These procedures permit in vivo examination of metabolic and/or neurotransmitter activation in the brain (see Roland, 1993). Figure 3.16 depicts a new method for imaging cholinergic activity in the hippocampus. These types of procedures are likely to lead to a mapping of neurotransmitter levels in the brain so that comparative studies can be performed. Additionally, the new procedures of functional magnetic resonance imaging (FMRI;

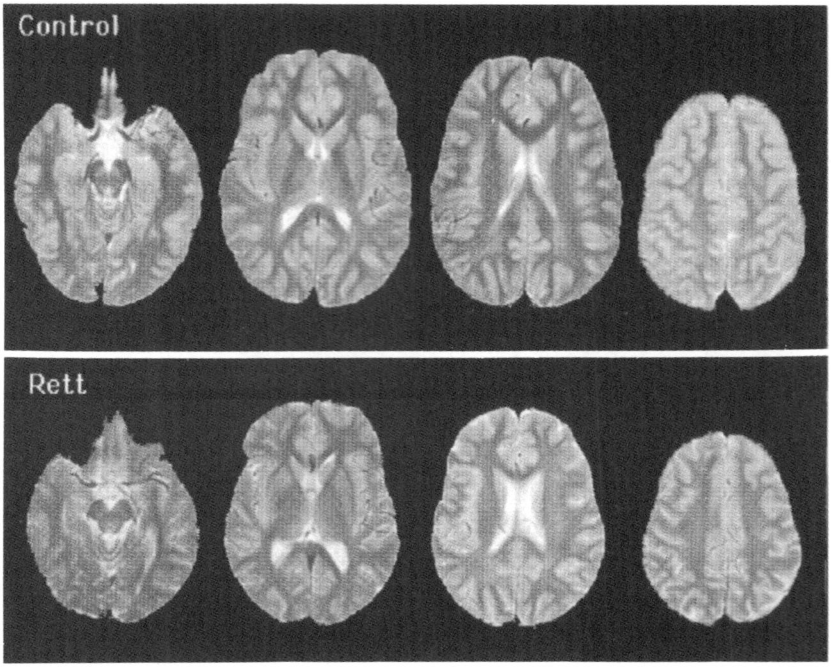

Fig. 3.14. At top: Representative control subject compared to (bottom) a Rett Syndrome child representative of the mean values obtained in the morphometric analysis of 14 control children and 9 children with Rett disorder. Table 3.3 presents the area measurement of the various ROIs. Notice that visual inspection of the Rett Syndrome case does not present with any marked or gross abnormality, but the comparing the size with that of the normal control based on the morphometric analysis indicates substantial differences between the two. Without such a morphometric and quantitative approach, Rett Syndrome scans have been interpreted as within normal limits. Quantitative neuroimaging data are presented in Table 3.3. (From Reiss, Faruque, Naidu, et al. (1993), by permission of *Annals of Neurology*. © Little, Brown & Co.)

Stehling, Turner, & Mansfield, 1991), and various new methods of quantitative electroencephalography (Gevins & Illes, 1991) hold great promise for enabling us to look at neuroimaging and functional outcome. In FMRI, an MR signal change occurs that is thought to relate to the deoxyhemoglobin concentration in specific regions of the brain microvasculature. Because of the magnetic properties of hemoglobin and focal increase of oxygenated blood during activation related to a specific brain region, FMRI may be capable of detecting differences in regional cerebral blood flow. Recently, Rao et al. (1993) have demonstrated functional imaging of complex motor movements using FMRI technology. The quantitative electroencephalography technique as discussed above by

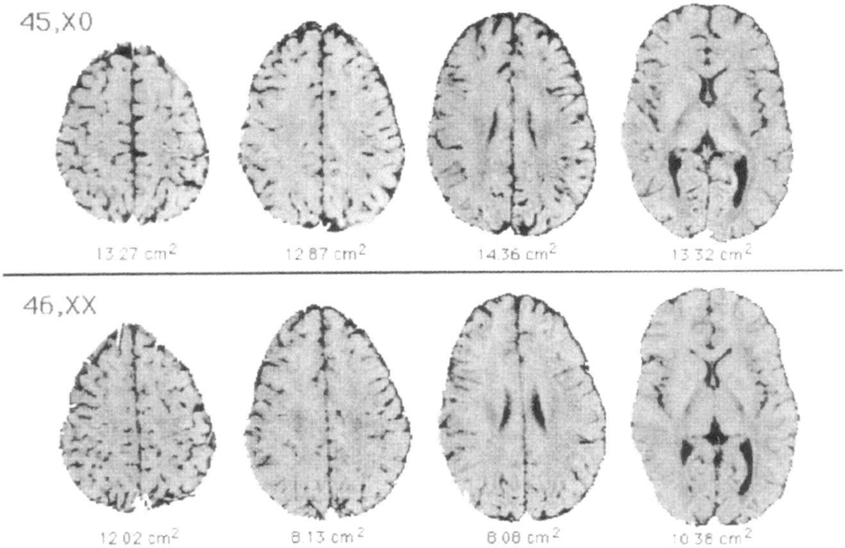

Fig. 3.15. Quantitative neuroanatomy of Turner's Syndrome by comparing a twin dysconcordant for the disorder. Table 3.4 presents the quantitative morphometric analysis of the two brains. Again, it is difficult to detect some of the differences between the two brains wherein one sibling has Turner's Syndrome and the other does not, but quantitative analysis certainly points toward some distinct anatomic differences. This anatomic information can then be compared to the neuropsychological outcome findings that are presented in Table 3.5. (From Reiss, Freund, Plotnick, et al. (1993), by permission of *Annals of Neurology*. © Little, Brown & Co.)

Table 3.3. Area measures (cm^2) determined from the midsagittal image.

Areas	Rett ($n = 9$) (mean ± SD)	Control ($n = 14$) (mean ± SD)	Rett/control (%)
Intracranial[a]	126.19 ± 8.56	154.29 ± 8.18	81.8
Cortical[a]	66.57 ± 5.14	90.15 ± 6.41	73.9
Corpus callosum[b]	5.15 ± 0.70	7.27 ± 0.97	70.8
Midbrain[b]	2.02 ± 0.26	2.72 ± 0.29	74.3
Pons[c]	4.82 ± 0.61	5.37 ± 0.53	89.8
4th ventricle	0.82 ± 0.20	1.00 ± 0.33	82.0
Vermis	10.81 ± 1.04	11.30 ± 1.38	95.7
Anterior vermis (lobules I–V)	4.41 ± 0.45	4.69 ± 0.61	94.0
Lobules VI and VII	3.14 ± 0.26	3.15 ± 0.48	99.7
Lobules VIII–X	3.26 ± 0.58	3.46 ± 0.64	94.2

[a] $p \leq 0.00005$ (one-tailed).
[b] $p \leq 0.0001$ (two-tailed).
[c] $p \leq 0.05$ (two-tailed).
SD = standard deviation.

Table 3.4. Quantitative neuroanatomy.

	TS (45,X)	(Adj)[a]	NS (46,XX)	TS (Adj)[a] % of NS
Total cerebral and hemispheric volumes[b]				
Total cerebrum	1,229.55	(1,187.09)	1,187.09	100
Total CSF	131.88	(127.33)	101.44	126
Rt hemisphere	612.67	(591.51)	597.29	99
Rt hemisphere CSF	63.60	(61.40)	48.96	125
Lt hemisphere	617.89	(596.55)	589.79	101
Lt hemisphere CSF	68.49	(66.13)	52.49	126
Total gray	637.72	(615.69)	643.76	96
Total white	459.94	(444.06)	441.88	100
Rt hemisphere gray	318.50	(307.50)	326.16	94
Rt hemisphere white	230.52	(222.56)	221.95	100
Lt hemisphere gray	319.81	(308.77)	317.61	97
Lt hemisphere white	229.70	(221.76)	219.93	101
	Twin TS (45,X)		**Twin NS (46,XX)**	**TS % of NS**
Midsagittal areas[c]				
Intracranial	151.49		149.26	102
Cortical	94.32		90.52	104
Corpus callosum	7.11		7.02	101
Ant vermis, lobules I–V	4.09		4.63	88
Post vermis, lobules VI, VII	2.06		2.73	75
Post vermis, lobules VIII–X	2.91		3.11	94
Posterior fossa[d]				
Medulla	4.02		4.52	89
Pons	10.98		12.97	85
Midbrain	9.06		8.33	108
Total brainstem (medulla, pons, midbrain)	24.07		25.82	92
Fourth vertricle	2.15		1.45	148
Third ventricle	0.39		0.31	126
Rt cerebellar hemisphere	64.40		59.91	108
Lt cerebellar hemisphere	62.62		61.52	102
Total cerebellum	127.03		121.43	105
Cisterna magna	9.24		6.01	154
Basal ganglia and lat ventricle[e]				
Rt caudate	5.08		4.87	104
Lt caudate	5.08		4.82	105
Rt putamen	6.19		6.09	102
Lt putamen	5.90		5.85	101
Rt globus pallidus	2.43		2.44	100
Lt globus pallidus	2.44		2.50	97
Rt lat ventricle	8.22		6.93	119
Lt lat ventricle	7.68		7.76	99

[a] Adjusted values for TS (in parentheses) are derived by multiplying the measured volumes for TS by 0.964 (NS total brain volume/TS total brain volume).
[b] Analyses were performed on composite images processed from 5-mm, contiguous, T2- and proton density-weighted scans in the axial plane. All values shown are volumes in cubic centimeters (cm^3).
[c] Analyses were performed on 3-mm midsagittal section. All values shown are areas in square centimeters (cm^2).
[d] Analyses were performed on 3-mm, contiguous, T1-weighted scans in the axial plane. All values shown are volumes in cubic centimeters (cm^3).
[e] Analyses were performed on 3-mm, contiguous, inversion recovery scans in the axial plane. All values shown are volumes in cubic centimeters (cm^3).
TS = twin with Turner's syndrome; NS = TS's sister; CSF = cerebrospinal fluid; Rt = right; Lt = left; Ant = anterior; Post = posterior; lat = lateral.

Gevins & Illes (1991), combined with MR anatomical precision, provide additional information about physiologic changes in brain function related to specific tasks. The potential of FMRI and quantitative electroencephalography is exciting and is discussed in greater detail in the next section.

Relevance of New Neuroimaging Methods for Select Clinical Syndromes

Attention Deficit Hyperactivity Disorder

Attention Deficit Hyperactivity Disorder (ADHD) remains one of the most prevalent neuropsychiatric disorders, but its etiology and underlying neurobiologic mechanisms are poorly understood (Hynd, Hern, Novey, Eliopulos, Marshal, Gonzalez, & Voeller, 1993). As far back as 1978, shortly after clinical introduction of CT scanning, Bergstrom and Bille reported that approximately one-third of a sample of children with so-called minimal brain dysfunction (MBD) had identifiable CT abnormalities. Shaywitz et al. (1983), however, did not find significant abnormalities in CT scanning in a select group of ADHD children when the CT findings were subjected to quantitative analysis and compared to matched controls. A year later, Lou et al. (1984; see also Lou, Henriksen, & Bruhn, 1989; Lou, Henriksen, Bruhn, Börner, & Nielsen, 1989) demonstrated that ADHD children demonstrated hypofusion on regional cerebral blood-flow studies. The Lou et al. study was the first to directly implicate neuroregulatory systems in the basal ganglia and frontal region of the brain, although it had long been speculated that such systems were related to the ADHD syndrome (Chelune, Ferguson, Koon, & Dickey, 1986; Mattes, 1980; Voeller, 1991). Despite these findings the early in 1980s, the picture that formed with additional studies in the latter part of that decade was clouded by confusion and inconsistent results.

More recent studies, focusing on magnetic-resonance imaging and careful quantitative methods, have yielded more positive and consistent results in ADHD. Hynd and colleagues (Hynd & Semrud-Clikeman, 1989; Hynd, Semrud-Clikeman, Lorys, Novey, & Eliopulos, 1990; Hynd, Semrud-Clikeman, Lorys, Novey, Eliopulos, Lyytinen, 1991; Hynd et al., Leonard et al., 1993) demonstrate greater likelihood of caudate nucleus asymmetry in ADHD children as well as differences in corpus callosum morphology. Hynd et al. interpret these findings as indicating potential anatomic irregularities that may underlie the physiologic aberration apparent in striatal-frontal systems. Zametkin et al. (1990) demonstrates that adults with a history of ADHD as children show decreased glucose metabolism in the brain, particularly in the prefrontal cortical region. The speculation has been that critical attentional systems may be under-

Table 3.5. Neuropsychological test results showing differences between the twins.

	Twin TX (45,X) standard score (percentile)	Twin NS (46,XX) standard score (percentile)
Psychoeducational testing domain		
Aptitude		
Wechsler Intelligence Scale for Children—Revised		
FSIQ	135 (99th)	145 (99th)
VIQ	143 (99th)	146 (99th)
PIQ	118 (88th)	136 (99th)
Factors		
Verbal Comprehension	144 (99th)	144 (99th)
Perceptual Comprehension	116 (86th)	137 (99th)
Achievement		
Woodcock-Johnson Psychoeducational Battery-Revised		
Tests of Achievement (W-J)		
Reading Cluster	126 (96th)	136 (99th)
Math Cluster	143 (99th)	140 (99th)
Written Expression Cluster	138 (99th)	139 (99th)

	(45,XO) raw scores	±SD from age (group mean)	(46,XX) raw scores	±SD from age (group mean)
Neuropsychological Subdomain				
Visual-Spatial Perception	37	40.6[a]	47	41.3[a]
Face Recognition total correct	8		14+	
Age equivalence (yr)				
Money Street Map	2	NA	0	NA
Forward direction errors	2, 18	NA	1, 09	NA
Forward direction time	15	NA	0	NA
(min, sec)	1, 47	NA	1, 19	NA
Toward self errors	17	12.8[a]	0	10.8[a]
Toward self time (min, sec)				
Total errors				

Visual-motor				
WISC-R Block design	15	1.7	18	2.7
WISC-R Object assembly	12	0.7	15	1.7
Rey-Osterrieth Figure Copy-inventory	26.5	−0.9	31.0	0.3
Visual memory				
Dot Localization total correct	15	−0.9	18	0.4
Self-regulation				
TOVA				
Omissions	0	−0.6	0	−0.6
Commissions	1	−1.5	3	−1.0
Mean reaction time (RT)	579	2.3	452	0.5
RT standard deviation	110	−0.7	69	−1.9
Executive Function				
Rey-Osterrieth organization score (total [age equivalent])				
Copy	6 (8 yr)	−0.7	13 (14+ yr)	1.2
Immediate recall	6 (8–9 yr)	−0.7	13 (14+ yr)	1.1
Delayed rccall	12 (14+ yr)	0.9	6 (8–9 yr)	−0.7
Word Fluency-Phonemic				
Total correct (percentile)	32 (80th)	NA	45 (>95th)	NA
Selective Reminding				
Consistent Long-Term Retrieval (CLTR)	30	−3.1	55	5.0
Ratio of CLTR/LTS	0.57	NA	1.00	NA

[a] Mean for age group. No norms available from which to calculate deviation from age-group mean in standard deviation units.
TS = twin with Turner's syndrome; NS = TS's sister; FSIQ = Full-Scale IQ; VIQ = Verbal IQ; PIQ = Performance IQ.

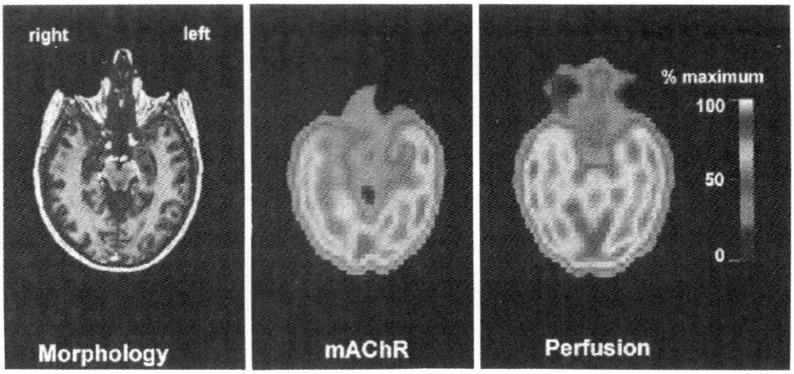

Fig. 3.16. Future applications of neuroimaging for neurotransmitter identification. Morphology, muscarinic acetylcholine receptor binding, and profusion in temporal lobe in patient with left-side temporal-lobe epilepsy. (a) MRI scan showing temporal-lobe morphology. A region-of-interest template, each region measuring 7 × 7 mm, was drawn on the MRI and transferred into the coregistered SPECT images for quantification. Regions were placed in the anterior hippocampus, amygdala, and temporal neocortex (three each—anterior, middle, and posterior temporal cortex). (b) Specific ^{123}I-Iododexetimide (^{123}I-IDex) binding was measured six to seven hours after tracer injection. Specific binding was computed as $(T - N)/N$, where T is the mean pixel value in a given temporal region and N the mean pixel values in the cerebellum indicating nonspecific binding. A pronounced reduction in specific ^{123}I-IDex binding in the anterior hippocampus ipsilateral to the electrical focuses is observed. A slight circumscribed reduction in the middle temporal neocortex, but no difference in other parts of the temporal lobe, was also seen (neuroSPECT, Summit Nuclear-Itachi; in-plane resolution 13.5 mm; z-axis resolution, 18 mm). (c) A slight reduction in cerebral profusion in the anterior temporal neocortex and left anterior hippocampus ipsilateral to the electrical focus compared with the contralateral side was seen (neuroSPECT).

activated, which would explain why stimulant or activation medications bring attentional abilities into a more optimal range.

These neuroanatomic studies have great promise for unraveling many of the abnormalities and irregularities that may attend the ADHD syndrome. It may be that some noninvasive neuroimaging tests, in conjunction with neuropsychological measures, will help in diagnosing ADHD and may provide the basis for better understanding this disorder. Various diagnostic classifications within the ADHD spectrum may also be more clearly defined by such methodologic approaches.

Learning Disorders

As already alluded to, several studies demonstrate various imaging irregularities in learning-disabled children (see Hynd & Semrud-Clikeman, 1989). This neuroimaging research follows Galaburda's contribution in demonstrating architectonic (Galaburda, Sherman, Rosen, Aboitiz, & Geschwind, 1985) and electrophysiologic (Livingstone, Rosen, Drislane, & Galaburda, 1991) factors in developmental dyslexia. Several recent quantitative MR studies continue to demonstrate abnormalities in the brain of children with reading disorder/dyslexia (Duara, Kush, Gross-Glenn, Barker, Jallad, Pascal, Loewenstein, Sheldon, Rabin, Levin, & Lubs, 1991; Jernigan, Hesselink, Sowell, & Tallal, 1991; Larsen, Hoien, Lundberg, & Odegaard, 1990; Leonard, Voeller, Lombardino, Morris, Hynd, Alexander, Anderson, Garofalakis, Honeyman, Mayo, Agge, & Stabb, 1993; Rumsey, Dorwart, Vermess, Denckla, Kruesi, & Rapoport, 1986; however, see Schultz et al., in press). Recently, we (Willerman, Schultz, Rutledge, & Bigler, 1991, 1992) and others (Andreasen, Flaum, Swayze, O'Leary, Alliger, Cohen, Earhardt, & Yuh, 1993) have demonstrated potential size factor differences in brain area that may relate to intellectual development. The convergence of this research suggests that anatomic parameters are likely to underlie some learning disorders and/or developmental delays that can be detected with neuroimaging technology (see Price, Deffner, Stowe, & Mesulam, 1990).

These research findings have potential widespread clinical importance. For example, most learning-disabled children are not seen for neuropsychological examination until somewhere past ages six to eight years. This is a time far beyond that of greatest brain plasticity. It may be that cerebral irregularities associated with learning disorder are identified earlier, intervention could take place during these more critical times. Research in this area will require close examination, combining developmental studies, brain imaging, and neuropsychological outcome.

Major Psychiatric Illnesses

The last two decades of neuroimaging research in psychiatric illness have greatly changed our understanding of neurobiologic factors that underlie so-called mental illnesses (Raz & Raz, 1990; Gillberg & Coleman, 1993). Nearly all major psychiatric illnesses, such as childhood autism, schizophrenia, affective disorder, and disorders of impulse control, have been investigated via the neuroimaging technique. Undoubtedly the one most widely researched is schizophrenia. It is now well understood that at least a subgroup of individuals with chronic schizophrenic illness have enlarged ventricles (Raz & Raz, 1990) and volume differences in frontal and temporal regions of the brain (Altshuler, Conrad, Hauser, Li, Guze, Denikoff, Tourtellotte, & Post, 1991; Andreasen, Nasrallah, Dunn, Olson, Grove, Ehrhardt, Coffman, & Crossett, 1986; Andreasen, Ehrhardt, Swayze, Alliger, Yuh, Cohen, & Ziebell, 1990). Research is now focusing, however, on specific nuclei such as the hippocampus, amygdala, and other limbic structures (Bartzokis, Mintz, Marx, Osborn, Gutkind, Chiang, Phelan, & Marder, 1993). These structures have long been thought to be involved in schizophrenic illness, but it has been difficult to study them in vivo. Current research is focused on establishing normative comparisons (Gur, Mozley, Resnick Shtasel, Kohn, Zimmerman, Herman, Atlas, Grossman, Erwin, & Gur 1991; Kohn, Tanna, Herman, Resnick, Mozley, Gur, Laavi, Zimmerman, & Gur, 1991) to compare to clinical subtypes (Bartzokis, Mintz, Marx, Osborn, Gutkind, Chiang, Phelan, & Marder, 1993). It is likely that future research in this area will provide additional insights into the neurobiology of major psychiatric illness, and we can hope it will lead to different options for treatment.

Future Directions

As described above, a number of new techniques are currently being applied, and they also form the basis for future implementation and clinical application in assessing childhood neurologic disorders. Brain imaging and neuropsychological assessment appears to have great promise. To conclude this chapter, I address and summarize several main areas from the previous discussions: standardizing of neuroimaging normative databases that are being developed with imaging technology, three-dimensional image display, functional MR imaging and spectroscopy, and early diagnostic imaging.

Standardization and Normative Data

Several recent articles deal with a comprehensive standardization approach to normal brain imaging (see Blatter et al., in press; Gur et al., 1991; Pfefferbaum et al., in press). As reviewed in this chapter, the initial research has focused on major structures such as brain, ventricular, and CSF volumes, along with large subcortical nuclei such as the corpus callosum, caudate nucleus, thalamus, and putamen, and some fiber track such as the fornix (Blatter et al., in press; Gale, Burr, Bigler, & Blatter, 1993). With current imaging resolution, however, even more refined analysis can be achieved. Damasio et al. (1991) demonstrate that MR imaging may capture regional cortical architecture. In the future it may be possible to study cellular layers of the cortex and more accurately follow interconnecting fiber tracks. This technology and standardization has very significant implications for detecting subtle cerebral asymmetries and anomalies that may be developmentally based, and it may lead to earlier diagnostic accuracy.

Three-Dimensional Image Analysis

Three-dimensional imaging has been discussed in this chapter, but looking into the future we can see much-increased application of the technique.

Real-time 3-D imaging will have a significant advantage over the current two-dimensional imaging analysis. With new, large computers that can adequately handle the data load, real-time motion and accurate volumetric assessment probably will become standard MR diagnostic approaches (see Damasio, Kulgis, Yuh, Van Hosesen, & Ehrhardt, 1991; Loftus, Tramro, Thomas, Green, Nordgren, & Gazzaniga, 1993). The quantitative normative database as discussed in this chapter is likely to be merged with 3-D image presentation to enhance accuracy in visualizing anatomic abnormality and how some pathologic states or shifts from normal relate to neuropsychological outcome.

Functional MR Imaging

Much has been learned about cerebral mechanisms of function by studying positron emission computed tomography (see Roland, 1993; Seitz, Roland, Bohm, Greitz, & Stone-Elanders, 1990). The problem with PET imaging, however, has been its inability to actieve refined image analysis (Posner, 1993). As introduced earlier, a promising technique is MR based—the so-called activation or functional MR (FMRI). With this technology the clinician in the future may be able to look directly at the brain with MR anatomic precision and measure blood-flow characteristics that can be used as direct in vivo measures of function. The implications are far-reaching. This method may provide online activation of aspects of blood-flow dynamics that can be significantly altered with a variety of disease/disorder state that also may relate systematically to cognitive and behavioral measurements. In the future, aspects of neuropsychological assessment may be performed directly with the patient in the MR scanner to simultaneously examine neuropsychological status, morphologically assess brain structure, and study functional activation patterns.

Spectroscopy

The MR spectroscopy (MRS) system applies MR methods to measuring metabolites in living tissue (see Keshavan, Kupur, & Pettegrew, 1991). These techniques have wide application for improved understanding of in vivo metabolic processes in the brain, neurotransmitter and neurotransmitter regulation, and effects of psychopharmacologic agents. Minshew et al. (1990) demonstrated membrane phospholipid activity levels between Alzheimers-disordered patients and Down syndrome. Similarly, Arnold et al. (1992) demonstrated consistent and diagnostically useful changes in spectroscopic findings in demyelinating brain lesions. Tzika et al. (1993) have used MR spectroscopy to assess a variety of neurodegenerative disorders. Combining MRS with FMRI has considerable clinical implications, especially that it will allow metabolic imaging with regional cerebral blood flow to be combined with the anatomic precision of standard MR.

Early Diagnostic Imaging

Huttenlocher et al. (1990) demonstrate several early behavioral measures that predict neurologic and neuropsychological outcome several years later. Developmental morphologic correlates might also be detected with imaging techniques as described above. Thus, developmental abnormalities might be detected at a much earlier age, as alluded to previously. Yokochi et al. (1991) demonstrate a relationship among several MR-identified abnormalities in children with spastic dyplesia and motor and mental outcome. Early diagnostic imaging might include even subtle developmental anomalies such as learning disorders. With improved functional and anatomical imaging of the brain, we will better understand the neurobiologic factors associated with the many newly recognized developmental disorders. The implications for recovering function and remediation are great. Kolb and Gibb (1991) demonstrate how an enriched environment facilitated aspects of neuroanatomical as well as behavioral recovery of function in a rodent model of TBI. If neuroimaging predictors of outcome can be determined and recognized early enough, they may guide therapeutic modalities during recovery.

Conclusion

Currently, neuroimaging can be approached quantitatively and the information can be integrated with neuropsychological evaluation. Nearly all neuroanatomic areas that can be identified with CT or MR technology can be volumetrically or morphometrically quantified. These quantitative data can be examined by comparison to normal or medical controls to determine the amount or degree of deviation from the norm. This neuroimaging information can then be compared to neuropsychological data, which also have been compared to a normative database. These comparisons provide an optimal circumstance for studying the anatomical basis for brain–behavior relationships. The next step is to focus on quantitative ways of integrating the neuroimaging and neuropsychological data to yield a single data format for presenting assessment findings in patients with some neurologic disorder.

References

Altshuler, L.L., Conrad, A., Hauser, P., Li, X., Guze, B.H., Denikoff, K., Tourtellotte, W., & Post, R. (1991). Reduction of temporal lobe volume in bipolar disorder: A preliminary report of magnetic resonance imaging. *Archives of General Psychiatry, 48,* 482–483.

Andreasen, N.C., Nasrallah, H.A., Dunn, V., Olson, S.C., Grove, W.M., Ehrhardt, J.C., Coffman, J.A., & Crossett, J.H. (1986). Structural abnormalities in the frontal system in schizophrenia: A magnetic resonance imaging study. *Archives of General Psychiatry, 43,* 136–144.

Andreasen, N.C., Ehrhardt, J.C., Swayze, V.W., Alliger, R.J., Yuh, W.T.C., Cohen, G., & Ziebell, S. (1990). Magnetic resonance imaging of the brain in schizophrenia: The path of physiologic significance of structural abnormalities. *Archives of General Psychiatry, 47,* 35–44.

Andreasen, N.C., Cizadlo, T., Harris, G., Swayze, V., O'Leary, D.S., Cohen, G., Earhardt, J., & Yuh, W.T.C. (1993). Voxel processing technique for the antemortem study of neuroanatomy and neuropathology using magnetic resonance imaging. *Journal of Neuropsychiatry, 5,* 121–130.

Andreasen, N.C., Flaum, M., Swayze, V., O'Leary, D.S., Alliger, R., Cohen, G., Earhardt, J., & Yuh, W.T.C. (1993). Intelligence and brain structure in normal individuals. *American Journal of Psychiatry, 150,* 130–134.

Arnold, D.L., Matthews, P.M., Francis, G.S., O'Connor, J., & Antel, J.P. (1992). Proton magnetic resonance spectroscopic imaging for metabolic characterization of demyelinating plaque. *Archives of Neurology, 31,* 235–241.

Barkovich, A.J. (1990). Apparent atypical callosal dysgenesis: Analysis of MR findings in six cases and their relationship to holoprosencephaly. *American Journal of Radiology, 153,* 127–134.

Barkovich, A.J., Chuang, S.H., & Norman, D. (1988). MR of neuronal migration anomalies. *American Journal of Radiology, 150,* 179–187.

Barkovich, A.J., & Norman, D. (1989). Absence of the septum pelucidum: A useful sign in the diagnosis of congenital brain malformation. *American Journal of Radiology, 152,* 353–360.

Barkovich, A.J., & Kjos, B.O. (1992a). Nonlissencephalic cortical dysplasias: Correlation of imaging findings with clinical deficits. *American Journal of Neuroradiology, 13,* 95–103.

Barkovich, A.J., & Kjos, B.O. (1992b). Schizencephaly: Correlation of clinical findings with MR characteristics. *American Journal of Neuroradiology, 13,* 85–94.

Bartzokis, G., Mintz, J., Marx, P., Osborn, D., Gutkind, D., Chiang, F., Phelan, C.K., & Marder, S.R. (1993). Reliability of in vivo volume measures of hippocampus and other brain structures using MRI. *Magnetic Resonance Imaging, 11,* 993–1006.

Bigler, E.D. (1988). The role of neuropsychological assessment in relation to other types of assessment with children. In M.G. Tramontana & S.R. Hooper (Eds.) (pp. 67–91). *Assessment issues in child neuropsychology.* New York: Plenum.

Bigler, E.D. (1990). *Traumatic brain injury.* Austin, TX: PRO-ED.

Bigler, E.D. (1991). Neuropsychological assessment neuroimaging in clinical neuropsychology: A synthesis. *Archives of Clinical Neuropsychology, 6,* 113–132.

Bigler, E.D. (1992a). The neurobiology and neuropsychology of adult learning disorders. *Journal of Learning Disabilities, 25,* 488–506.

Bigler, E.D. (1992b). Three-dimensional image analysis of trauma induced degenerative changes: An aid to neuropsychological assessment. *Archives of Clinical Neuropsychology, 7,* 449–456.

Bigler, E.D., Kurth, S., Blatter, D., & Abildskov, T. (1993). Day-of-injury CT as an index to pre-injury brain morphology: Degree of post-injury degenerative changes identified by CT and MR neuroimaging. *Brain Injury, 7,* 125–134.

Blatter, D., Bigler, E.D., Gale, S., Johnson, S., Anderson, C., Burnett, B., Kurth, S., & Horn, S. (1994). Quantitative neuroimaging: Normative MR database spanning five decades (pp. 16–65). *American Journal of Neuroradiology.*

Chelune, G.J., Ferguson, W., Koon, R., & Dickey, T.O. (1986). Frontal lobe disinhibition in attention deficit disorder. *Child Psychiatry and Human Development, 16,* 221–233.

Damasio, H., Kulgis, R.O., Yuh, Y., Van Hosesen, G.W., & Ehrhardt, J. (1991). Magnetic resonance imaging of human intracortical structures in vivo. *Cerebral Cortex, 1,* 374–379.

Damasio, H., & Frank, R. (1992). Three-dimensional in vivo mapping of brain lesion in humans. *Archives of Neurology, 49,* 137–143.

Duara, R., Kush, C.A., Gross-Glenn, K., Barker, W.W., Jallad, B., Pascal, S., Loewenstein, D.A., Sheldon, J., Rabin, M., Levin, B., & Lubs, H. (1991). Neuroanatomic differences between dyslexic and normal readers on magnetic resonance imaging scans. *Archives of Neurology, 48,* 410–416.

Eisenberg, R.L. (1992). *Radiology: An illustrated history.* St. Louis: Mosby Yearbook.

Galaburda, A.M., Sherman, G.F., Rosen, G.D., Aboitiz, F., & Geschwind, N. (1985). Developmental dyslexia: Four consecutive patients with cortical anomalies. *Annals of Neurology, 18,* 222–233.

Gale, S.D., Burr, R.B., Bigler, E.D., & Blatter, D. (1993). Fornix degeneration in memory and traumatic brain injury. *Brain Research Bulletin, 32,* 345–349.

Gevins, A.S., & Illes, J. (1991). Neurocognitive network of the human brain. *Annals of the New York Academy of Sciences, 620,* 22–44.

Gillberg, C., & Coleman, M. (1993). *The biology of the autistic syndrome* (2nd ed.). New York: Cambridge University Press.

Gur, R.E., Mozley, P.D., Resnick, S.M., Shtasel, D., Kohn, M., Zimmerman, R.A., Herman, G.T., Atlas, S., Grossman, R., Erwin, R., & Gur, R.C. (1991). Magnetic resonance imaging in schizophrenia: I. Volumetric analysis of brain and cerebral spinal fluid. *Archives of General Psychiatry, 48,* 407–412.

Heaton, R.L., Grant, I., & Matthews, C.G. (1992). *Comprehensive norms for an expanded Halstead-Reitan Battery: Demographic corrections, research findings, and clinical applications.* Odessa, FL: Psychological Assessment Resources.

Huttenlocher, P.R., Levine, S.C., Huttenlocher, J., & Gates, J. (1990). Discrimination of normal and at-risk preschool children on the basis of neurologic tests. *Developmental medicine and Child Neurology, 32,* 394–402.

Hynd, G.W., Semrud-Clikeman, M. (1989). Dyslexia and brain morphology. *Psychological Bulletin, 106,* 447–482.

Hynd, G.W., Semrud-Clikeman, M., Lorys, A.R., Novey, E.S., & Eliopulos, D. (1990). Brain morphology in developmental dyslexia and attention deficit disorder/hyperactivity. *Archives of Neurology, 47,* 919–926.

Hynd, G.W., Semrud-Clikeman, M., Lorys, A.R., Novey, E.S., Eliopulos, D., & Lyytinen, A. (1991). Corpus callosum morphology in attention deficit-hyperactivity disorder: Morphometric analysis of the MRI. *Journal of Learning Disabilities, 24,* 141–146.

Hynd, G.W., Hern, K.L., Novey, E.S., Eliopulos, D., Marshal, R., Gonzalez, J.J., & Voeller, K. K. (1993). Attention deficit-hyperactivity disorder and asymmetry of the caudate nucleus. *Journal of Child Neurology, 8,* 339–347.

Jernigan, T. L., Hesselink, J.R., Sowell, E., & Tallal, P.A. (1991). Cerebral structure on magnetic resonance imaging in language- and learning-impaired children. *Archives of Neurology, 48,* 539–547.

Keshaven, M.S., Kupur, S., & Pettegrew, J.W. (1991). Magnetic resonance spectroscopy in psychiatry: Potential, pitfalls, and promise. *American Journal of Psychiatry, 148,* 976–985.

Kim, S.G., Ashe, J., Hendrich, K., Ellermann, J.M., Merkle, H., Gurbil, K., & Georgopoulos, A.P. (1993). Functional magnetic resonance imaging of motor cortex: Hemispheric asymmetry in handedness. *Science, 261,* 615–617.

Kjos, B.O., Umansky, R., & Barkovich, A.J. (1990). Brain MR imaging in children with developmental retardation of unknown cause: Results in 76 cases. *American Journal of Neuroradiology, 11,* 1035–1042.

Kohn, M.I., Tanna, N.K., Herman, G.T., Resnick, S.M., Mozley, P.D., Gur, R.E., Laavi, A., Zimmerman, R.A., & Gur, R.C. (1991). Analysis of brain and CSF volumes from magnetic resonance images: Methodology, reliability and validation. *Radiology, 178,* 115–122.

Kolb, B., & Gibb, R. (1991). Environmental enrichment in cortical injury: Behavioral and anatomical consequences of frontal cortex lesions. *Cerebral Cortex, 1,* 189–198.

Larsen, J.P., Hoien, T., Lundberg, I., & Odegaard, H. (1990). MRI evaluation of the size and symmetry of the planum temporale in adolescents with developmental dyslexia. *Brain and Language, 39,* 289–301.

Leonard, C.M., Voeller, K.K.S., Lombardino, L.J., Morris, M.K., Hynd, J.W., Alexander, A.W., Andersen, H.G., Garofalakis, M., Honeyman, J.C., Mao, J., Agge, O.F., & Staab, E.V. (1993). Anomalous cerebral structure in dyslexia revealed with magnetic resonance imaging. *Archives of Neurology, 50,* 461–469.

Livingstone, M.S., Rosen, G.D., Drislane, F.W., & Galaburda, A.M. (1991). Physiological and anatomical evidence for a magnocellular defect in developmental dyslexia. *Proceedings of the National Academy of Science, 88,* 7943–7947.

Loftus, W.C., Tramro, M.J., Thomas, C.E., Green, R.L., Nordgren, R.A., & Gazzaniga, M.S. (1993). 3-dimensional quantitative analysis of hemispheric asymmetry in the human superior temporal region. *Cerebral Cortex, 3,* 348–355.

Lou, H.C., Henriksen, L., & Bruhn, P. (1984). Focal cerebral hypoperfusion in children with dysphasia and/or attention deficit disorder. *Archives of Neurology, 41,* 825–829.

Lou, H.C., Henriksen, L., & Bruhn, P. (1989). Striatal dysfunction in attention deficit and hyperkinetic disorder. *Archives of Neurology, 46,* 48–52.

Lou, H.C., Henriksen, L., Bruhn, P., Börner, H., & Nielsen, J.B. (1989). Striatal dysfunction in attention deficit and hyperkinetic disorder. *Archives of Neurology, 46,* 48–52.

Mattes, J.A. (1980). The role of frontal lobe function in childhood hyperkinesis. *Comprehensive Psychiatry, 21,* 358–369.

Minshew, W.J., Pettegrew, J.W., & Panchalingham, K. (1990). Membrane phospholipid alterations observed in Alzheimers disease are not present in Down's syndrome. *Biological Psychiatry, 27* (Suppl. 9A), 123–124.

Müller-Gärtner, H.W., Mayberg, H.S., Fisher, R.S., Lesser, R.P., Wilson, A.A., Ravert, H.T., Dannals, R.F., Wagner, H.N., Uematsu, S., & Frost, J.J. (1993). Decreased hippocampal muscarinic cholinergic receptor binding measured by ^{123}I-Iododexetimide & Single Photon. *Annals of Neurology, 34,* 235–238.

Oldendorf, W.H. (1980). *The quest for an image of brain.* New York: Raven Press.

Peterson, B., Riddle, M.A., Cowen, D.J., Katz, L.D., Smith, J.C., Hardin, M.T., & Leckman, J.F. (1993). Reduced basal ganglia volumes in Tourett's Syndrome using three-dimensional reconstruction techniques from magnetic resonance images. *Annals of Neurology.*

Pfefferbaum, A., Mathalon, D.H., Sullivan, E.V., Rawles, J.M., Zipursky, R.B., & Lim, K.O. (in press). A quantitative MRI study of changes in brain morphology from infancy to adulthood. *Archives of Neurology.*

Posner, M.I. (1993). Seeing the mind. *Science, 262,* 673–674.

Price, B.H., Daffner, K.R., Stowe, R.M., & Mesulam, M.M. (1990). The comportmental learning disabilities of early frontal damage. *Brain, 113,* 1383–1393.

Pujol, J., Vandrell, P., Junque, C., MartíVilalta, J.L., & Capdevila, A. (1993). When does human brain development end? Evidence of corpus callosum growth up to adulthood. *Annals of Neurology, 34,* 71–75.

Rao, S.M., Binder, J.R., Bandettini, P.A., Hammeke, T.A., Yetkin, F.Z., Jesmanowiz, A., Lisk, L.M., Morris, G.L., Mueller, W.M., Estkowski, L.D., Wong, E.C., Haughton, V.M., & Hyde, J.S. (1993). Functional magnetic resonance imaging of complex human movement. *Neurology, 43,* 2311–2318.

Raz, S., & Raz, N. (1990). Structural brain abnormalities in the major psychoses: A quantitative review of the evidence from computerized imaging. *Psychological Bulletin, 108,* 93–108.

Reiss, A.L., Faruque, F., Naidu, S., Abrams, M., Beaty, T., Bryan, R.N., & Moser, H. (1993a). Neuroanatomy of Rett Syndrome: A volumetric imaging study. *Annals of Neurology, 34,* 227–234.

Reiss, A.L., Freund, L., Plotnick, L., Baumgardner, T., Green, K., Sozer, A.C., Reader, M., Boehm, C., & Denckla, M.B. (1993b). The effects of X monosomy on brain development: Monozygotic twins discordant for Turner's Syndrome. *Annals of Neurology, 34,* 95–107.

Robb, R.A. (1990). A software system for interactive and quantitative analysis of biomedical images. In K.H. Höhne, H. Fuchs, & S.M. Pizer (Eds.), *3-D Imaging in Medicine,* NATO ASI Series, Vol. F60: 333–361.

Roland, P.E. (1993). *Brain activation.* New York: Wiley-Liss.

Rumsey, J.M., Dorwart, R., Vermess, M., Denckla, M.B., Kruesi, J.P.M., & Rapoport, J.L. (1986). Magnetic resonance imaging of brain anatomy in severe developmental dyslexia. *Archives of Neurology, 43,* 1045–1046.

Schultz, R.T., Cho, N.K., Staib, L.H., Kier, L.E., Fletcher, J.M., Shaywitz, S.E., Shankweiler, D.P., Katz, L., Gore, J.C., Duncan, J.S., & Shaywitz, B.A. (in press). Brain morphology in normal and dyslexic children: The influence of sex and age. *Archives of Neurology.*

Seitz, R.J., Roland, P.E., Bohm, C., Greitz, T., & Stone-Elanders, S. (1990). Motor learning in man: A positron emission tomography study. *Neuro Report, 1,* 117–119.

Shaywitz, B.A., Shaywitz, S.E., Byrne, T., Cohen, D.J., & Rothman, S. (1983). Attention deficit disorder: Quantitative analysis of CT. *Neurology, 33,* 1500–1503.

Stehling, N.K., Turner, R., & Mansfield, P. (1991). Echo-planer imaging: Magnetic resonance imaging in a fraction of a second. *Science, 254,* 43–54.

Turkheimer, E. (1989). Techniques of quantitative measurement of morphological structures of the central nervous system. In E.D. Bigler, R.A. Yeo, & E. Turkheimer (Eds.), *Neuropsychological function and brain imaging*. New York: Plenum Press.

Turkheimer, E., Cullum, C.M., Hubler, D.W., Paver, S.W., Yeo, R.A., & Bigler, E.D. (1984). Quantifying cortical atrophy. *Journal of Neurology, Neurosurgery and Psychiatry, 47,* 1314–1318.

Turkheimer, E., Yeo, R.A., & Bigler, E.D. (1990). Basic relations among lesion location, lesion volume and neuropsychological performance. *Neuropsychologia, 28,* 1011–1019.

Turkheimer, E., Yeo, R.A., Jones, C.L., & Bigler, E.D. (1990). Quantitative assessment of covariation between neuropsychological function and location of naturally occurring lesions in humans. *Journal of Clinical and Experimental Neuropsychology, 12,* 549–565.

Tzika, A.A., Ball, W.S., Vigneron, D.B., Dun, R.S., & Kirks, D.R. (1993). Clinical proton MR spectroscopy of neurodegenerative disease in childhood. *American Journal of Neuroradiology, 14,* 1267–1281.

Voeller, K.K.S. (1991). What can neurological models of attention, inattention, and arousal tell us about attention-deficit hyperactivity disorder? *Journal of Neuropsychiatry, 3,* 209–216.

Willerman, L., Schultz, R., Rutledge, J.N., & Bigler, E.D. (1991). In vivo brain size and intelligence. *Intelligence, 15,* 223–228.

Willerman, L., Schultz, R., Rutledge, J.N., & Bigler, E.D. (1992). Hemisphere size asymmetry predicts relative verbal and non-verbal intelligence differently in the sexes: An MRI study of structure-function relation. *Intelligence, 16,* 315–328.

Wolpert, S.M., & Barnes, P.D. (1992). *MRI in Pediatric Neuroradiology,* St. Louis: Mosby Yearbook.

Yokochi, K., Aiba, K., Hori, E.M., Inukai, K., Fujimoto, S., Kodama, M., & Kodama, K. (1991). Magnetic resonance imaging in children with spastic diplegia: Correlation with the severity of their motor and mental abnormality. *Child Neurology-Developmental Medicine, 33,* 18–25.

Zametkin, A.J., Nordahl, T.E., Gross, M., King, A.C., Semple, W.E., Rumsey, J., Hamburger, S., & Cohen, R.M. (1990). Cerebral glucose metabolisms in adults with hyperactivity of childhood onset. *New England Journal of Medicine, 323,* 1361–1390.

CHAPTER 4

A Test-Profile Approach in Analyzing Cognitive Disorders in Children: Experiences of the NEPSY

MARIT KORKMAN

Background to the Development of the NEPSY

Throughout the western countries, clinical neuropsychology has become established as a basic part of the treatment of neurological patients and children with learning disorders. In one area, however, cultural and lingual differences may obstruct the flow of new advances across borders—the spreading of new tests.

Tests need to be elaborated in the appropriate language and they must also be standardized on a representative national sample. For small nations and populations, standardizing tests is economically possible only for those most commonly used, such as the Wechsler Scales. The problem is most critical in tests for children, which need separate test norms for each age level. Furthermore, assessing children relies heavily on test norms, because what is normal or subnormal for children is highly age dependent.

In Finland, the only tests amenable to child neuropsychology that have had national norms have been the Wechsler Intelligence Scales for Children-Revised (WISC-R; Wechsler, 1984) and the Illinois Test of Psycholinguistic Abilities (ITPA; Kuusinen & Blåfield, 1974). Other tests were used, though Finnish norms were lacking, by referring to American norms. Such tests included the Wechsler Primary and Preschool Scales of Intelligence (WPPSI; Wechsler, 1977), the Developmental Test of Visuo-Motor Integration (VMI; Beery & Buktenica, 1967), the Token Test (DeRenzi & Vignolo, 1962), the Motor-Free Visual Perception Test (MVPT; Colarusso & Hammill, 1972), the Rey-Ostereith Figure (Lezak, 1983), and techniques described by Benton et al. (1983). The Halstead-Reitan and Reitan-Indiana batteries (Reitan, 1979) were not widely used in Finland.

Luria's methods, as presented by his pupil Maruszewski (1971) and by Christensen (1975, 1984), were commonly practiced with adult patients. An experimental version for children age 5 and 6 was also developed and standardized (Korkman, 1980). This adaptation of Luria's method for children differed from that of Golden (1987) by keeping the subtests separate instead of creating sum scores. One shortcoming of the method was the narrow age range of the norms. Another was that the tests were of pass-fail type, which did not correspond to the developmental variability of children's abilities. The comprehensiveness of the method as well as the application of Luria's approach to children were appreciated, however, and led to the endeavor of integrating this approach with prevalent psychometric traditions of child neuropsychology.

Previous child neuropsychological assessments and tests were reviewed, and a collection of tests was further elaborated and standardized. The new assessment was called NEPSU, an acronym for the Finnish name (Korkman, 1988a, 1988b, 1988c, 1990a). A corresponding version, NEPSY, was soon published in Swedish (Korkman, 1990b). Subsequently, the method is called NEPSY (from NEuroPSYchological Investigation for Children).

In this chapter we present the NEPSY together with experiences and findings obtained with this assessment. The description of the NEPSY may be of interest internationally, for an American adaptation is being developed (Korkman, Kirk, & Kemp, in press).

The Finnish and the Swedish versions differ in some respects, the former being standardized for a broader age range (4 to 8 years) than the latter (4 to 7 years). Below, the Finnish version will be described unless otherwise specified.

The NEPSY

Rationales for the Assessment

One main requirement of a neuropsychological assessment is that it be comprehensive and cover the main types of functions that may be affected in various kinds of developmental and acquired brain disorders. The tradition in child neuropsychology has been to evaluate these domains: attention, language, executive and motor skills, perception, spatial construction, and memory (Mattis, 1992). These areas were also the targets for the NEPSY.

A second requirement of the assessment was that the tests allow for analyzing the nature and mechanisms of cognitive and psychomotor disorders. The tests should therefore assess many discrete functions rather than a few broad constructs. Luria's investigation (Christensen, 1975) was an important model in this respect.

Luria's investigation is directed toward qualitative analysis of complex cognitive disorders by clarifying the nature and mechanisms of the disorders. In his theory, Luria specifies the main subprocesses or components of complex functions such as speech, memory, perception, and manual skills. The components of these areas are represented in the neuropsychological investigation in the form of carefully targeted tests. For example, language is assessed by testing phonemic analysis, comprehension of words, sentences, and syntactic structures, articulation, repetition, naming, and narrative speech. The results are interpreted by specifying the primary deficiencies of a disorder. The primary deficiency of an aphasia, for example, may be impaired phonemic coding of speech. The interpretation may be verified by formulating and testing hypotheses about the expected secondary consequences (Christensen, 1975, 1984; Luria, 1973, 1980; see also pp. 95–97).

Luria's principles of neuropsychological analysis of cognitive disorders are not unique. They employ principles inherent in most neuropsychological diagnostic efforts, not only when assessing adult patients, but also when analyzing children's cognitive disorders. For example, Pennington (1991) distinguishes primary, secondary, and correlated symptoms in learning-disordered children. Wilson (1992) advocates a construct-driven assessment by evaluating deficits or constructs in a flexible, hypothesis-testing way.

Luria's methods for localizing brain damage were, however, not directly applicable to learning-disordered children, because the mechanisms of learning disorders may differ from those of cognitive disorders after acute brain injury in adults. Nor did the pass/fail format of Luria's tests correspond to the psychometric traditions of most tests for children.

The general aim in constructing the assessment was thus to assemble and psychometrically evolve tests that would cover the main components of cognitive functions that are frequently impaired in children. As many as thirty-eight tests were drafted, based on the traditions of child neuropsychological assessment (e.g., Benton, Hamsher, Varney, & Spreen, 1983; Rourke, Bakker, Fisk, & Strang, 1983; Rourke, Fisk, & Strang, 1986), Luria's investigation (Christensen, 1975; Maruszewski, 1971), and other neuropsychological procedures used with adult patients (e.g., Lezak, 1983).

Many of the developed tests were thus adaptations or new versions of previous test ideas, which were reformulated to provide approximately the same format for all tests. Other tests were new or resembled earlier tests only by being targeted toward a specific function. Two tests, the shortened version of the Token Test (DeRenzi & Faglioni, 1978) and the VMI (Beery, 1983; Beery & Buktenica, 1967), were added to the assessment in their original form and were standardized together with the new tests. In the Swedish version several additional tests also were standardized, among these the MVPT (Colarusso & Hammill, 1972) and a Swedish test of visual perception (Borg, 1977). These tests were seen as complements to, rather than parts of, the NEPSY, but because they were standardized along with the NEPSY tests they could be utilized in interpreting the test profile.

One requirement for the format was that the tests be developmentally sensitive and capable of reflecting developmental changes and subtle deficiencies. This requirement was best met by constructing the tests as psychometric, homogeneous scales with test items of increasing difficulty, and by developing separate norms for various age levels (Anastasi, 1982; Cronbach, 1984). The target age range was set at 4 to 8 years, because probably most children sent to neuropsychological assessments in Finland are recruited from this age group.

To permit comparison of the test results in one profile they also had to be simultaneously standardized. Separately collected test norms may vary depending on sampling procedures, and they also tend to grow obsolete. A test profile based on separately standardized tests may therefore reflect properties of the test norms, and not just an individual's strengths and weaknesses (Russell, 1986; Wilson, 1992). Simultaneously developed and standardized tests would permit psychometrically valid intraindividual comparison of areas of performance; that is, a test-profile approach. Consequently, a wide range of tests was included. It was reasoned that tests could later be dropped if not shown to be valid, whereas tests could not be added after the standardization.

The NEPSY Tests

The NEPSY consists of five main parts: (1) tests of attention, orientation, and application of strategy in executing performances, (2) language tests, (3) sensory-motor tests, (4) visual-spatial tests, and (5) tests of memory and learning. Each part includes several separate tests that are designed to represent the main components of the broader areas of functioning.

Tests of Orientation, Attention, and Strategy

General Orientation. The child is asked questions about time and place as well as personal data (e.g., birthdate, address; cf. Wechsler Memory Scale (WMS); Christensen, 1975).

Inhibition and Control. Five tasks are presented, in which the child is required to control impulses. In one of the tasks the child should sit with eyes closed and resist opening them in spite of the examiner's knocking on the table, or bringing a ticking clock close to the child's ear (adapted from Benton et al., 1983). In two other tasks the child should do the opposite of what the examiner does, such as knock on the table when the examiner taps and tap when the examiner knocks (Christensen, 1975). A fourth task requires the child to stand still "like a soldier on guard" (adapted from Manuilenko, 1975). In the fifth task the examiner says, in a long sequence, *door, ceiling, floor, ceiling* . . . The child is instructed to point to the door when hearing the word *door*, point to the floor when hearing the word *floor*, but not to point when hearing the word *ceiling*.

Verbal Fluency. In the NEPSY version of the word fluency test the child is to name as many animals and as many things to eat or drink as he or she can think of in a minute (cf. Isaacs & Kennie, 1973; McArthy Scales of Children's Abilities (McArthy, 1972; Spreen & Strauss, 1991).

Sustained Concentration. The test consists of the average time the child is able to keep working continuously during the testing sessions (maximum 45 minutes).

Selective Auditory Attention. A five-minute sequence of words is read to the child in a monotonous voice. Each time the word *red* is pronounced the child is to pick a red peg from a box of colored pegs and put it in a pegboard. The test's length, monotony, and infrequent demand for reactions make it invite lapses in attention.

The Sorting Test. This test is similar to the Wisconsin Card Sorting test (Berg, 1948), but simpler. Four cards are placed before the child: a yellow circle, a red star, a blue triangle, and a green cross. A pack of similar cards is presented, one card at a time, and the child is to point either to a similar color or a similar shape on one of the initial cards. One of these sorting principles is reinforced until six correct consecutive sortings are achieved, after which the sorting principle is changed without informing the child. Successful performance requires the capacity to deduce the sorting principle from the reinforcement provided and adjust responses accordingly.

Language Tests

Auditory Analysis of Speech. This test consists of sound-blending and word-completion tasks. The child responds by pointing out the correct picture among three alternatives. In English a sound-blending task could be, "Here you see children, chicken, and a kitchen. Now point to *ki-tchen*." A word-completion task could be, "Here you see a castle, a postcard, and candy. In which word is there a part such as *-ost*?" (cf. ITPA).

Comprehension of Instructions. In this paper-and-pencil test the child is to follow verbal instructions, such as *Draw a circle in the middle of the paper!* and *Draw two lines, one on each side of the circle!*

The Token Test. The shortened version by DeRenzi and Faglioni (1978) is included as a complementary test. The child is required to follow verbal instructions of varying length and complexity by pointing out or manipulating tokens. Examples of the instructions are: *Point to a yellow square and a black square!* and *Put the red circle on top of the green square!*

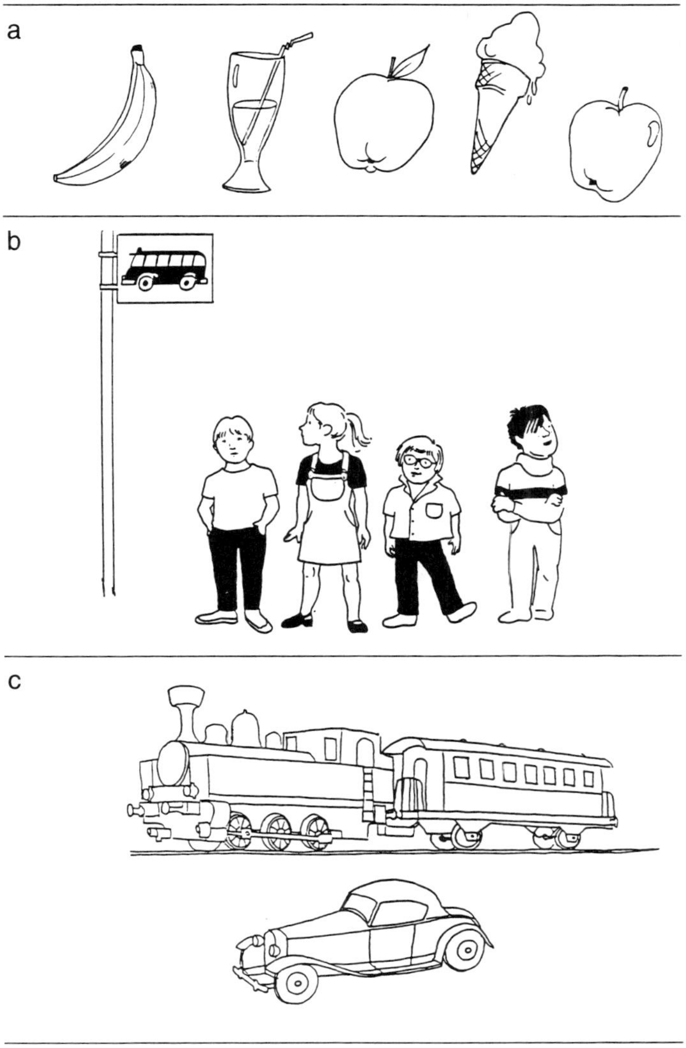

Fig. 4.1. Examples of tasks from the Relative Concepts test. The child is to point out the appropriate picture when asked: What is between the apples? (a); Which child is beside the bus stop? (b); If this train goes faster than that car, which one goes slower? (c).

Relative Concepts. The child is to demonstrate comprehension of verbal-logical concepts and relations by pointing out specific pictures. Examples include the thing that is *between the apples* or *the child who is beside the bus stop*. A more demanding item is, *If this train goes faster than that car, which one goes slower?* (Figure 4.1) (adapted from Boehm, 1969, 1971; Christensen, 1975; Maruszewski, 1971).

Comprehension of Syntactic Cues. The child is asked questions such as, *Can a mother be taken care of by her baby?* (in the Swedish version).

Oral Kinesthetic Praxis. The child is to imitate positions and movements of the oral apparatus, such as pushing the cheek with the tongue, putting the lower lip over the upper lip, and to articulate some difficult sounds, such as *rrr*, *ssss*, and *schhhh* (cf. Christensen, 1975; Lezak, 1983; Maruszewski, 1971).

Oral Dynamic Praxis. The child is asked to repeat ten times phonological sequences or tongue-twisters. In English, one sequence could be, *scoobelly doobelly/scoobelly doobelly* (cf. Christensen, 1975; Maruszewski, 1971).

Repeating Words and Nonwords. The child is to repeat phonologically complex words, such as *screwdriver*, and nonwords, such as *asjection* (cf. Christensen, 1975; Maruszewski, 1971; Spreen & Benton, 1965; Spreen & Strauss, 1991).

Naming Colors. The child is to name the colors of seven color samples (cf. Griffiths' scales) (Alin-Åkerman & Nordberg, 1980; Christensen, 1975; Maruszewski, 1971).

Naming Body Parts. Nine body parts are pointed out in pictures and the child is asked to name them (cf. Christensen, 1975; Maruszewski, 1971).

Naming Tokens. The child is to name, as quickly as possible, the size, color, and shape of pictures of the 20 tokens from the Token Test. Both the number of errors and the performance time are recorded (adapted from Vilkki & Laitinen, 1974).

Storytelling. A story is told to the child, after which the child should tell all he or she remembers of the content. Both number and order of elements are scored. To evaluate the capacity to formulate the story, the test score is contrasted to that of cued memory for the story (cf. Christensen, 1975).

Reading Readiness. This test measures preliminary skills of the preschool child in reading and spelling, and consists of tasks of letter knowledge, extracting the beginning phonemes in words, and reading syllables. The test is not intended to measure achievement in reading and spelling.

Sensory-Motor Tests

Handedness. The test consists of six tasks of handedness, including drawing, erasing, pricking holes in a paper with a pin, and so on (cf. Annett, 1970; Auzias, 1975).

Kinesthetic Praxis—Position of Hands. The child imitates positions of the hand, such as putting the thumb between the middle finger and the ring finger, or pointing outward with the thumb and the little finger while keeping the other fingers in a fist (adapted from Christensen, 1975).

Dynamic Praxis—Manual Movement Series. The child is taught manual motor series and tries to repeat them ten times in a sequence. One task is to clap the hands, tap the palms on the table, clap, tap, and so on. Another task: right-hand knuckles knock on the table, left-hand knuckles knock on the table, right-hand palm taps, left-hand palm taps (adapted from Christensen, 1975; Maruszewski, 1971).

Kinesthetic Feedback from Positions. The child stands on the floor, eyes closed. The examiner puts one of the child's arms in a position, such as straight out with fingers extended. The child is to put the other arm in the mirror position. Tasks are performed with both the right and the left arm (cf. Alahuhta, 1978).

Kinesthetic Feedback from Movements. The examiner draws letters and figures in the air with the child's hand and child sitting with eyes closed. The child is to tell which letter (O, V, S) or which figure (a ball, a point, or a rope) is drawn, each time. The tasks are performed with both hands.

Tactile Perception of Forms. The same letters and figures as above are drawn by the examiner with the tip of the finger on the child's palm, child sitting with eyes closed. Tasks are presented for both hands (adapted from Rey, 1964).

Tactile Finger Discrimination. The child's hand is shielded from his or her sight by a sheet of paper. The examiner touches one finger at a time. The child is to tell which finger was touched or to point to the appropriate finger upon lifting the shield. The task is performed on both hands (adapted from Benton, Hamsher, Varney, & Spreen, 1983).

Left-Right Difference. The scores for the right and the left hand in the four tests above are calculated and compared (cf. Reitan, 1979).

Visuo-Motor Precision. In this paper-and-pencil test the child is to draw a continuous line on a curvilinear route without crossing its borders (Frostig, Lefever, & Whittlesey, 1963).

Visual-Spatial Tests

Slopes of Lines. The test material consists of pictures in which the child is to point out which arrows point to a target (cf. Benton, Varney, & Hamsher, 1975).

Block Construction. The child is to build constructions with blocks after models in pictures. If the child fails in a task, the construction is demonstrated (cf. McCarthy, 1972; Terman & Merrill, 1973).

Venger's Map Test. The child is to find a route to a target on a map according to directions indicated by drawings of the route (adapted from Venger & Holmomskaya, 1978).

Left-Right Orientation. The child is asked to indicate his or her left hand, right ear, and left knee (cf. Benton, Hamsher, Varney, & Spreen, 1983).

Neglect. The child is to put a pencil mark at the midpoints of lines on a sheet (cf. Diller, Ben-Yishay, Gerstman, Goodkin, Gordon, & Weinberg, 1974).

The VMI (Beery, 1983; Beery & Buktenica, 1967). This test is a complement to the NEPSY test. The tasks consist of copying geometric designs.

Tests of Memory and Learning

Digit Span. The test consists of repeating progressively longer digit series forward (cf. WISC-R; WMS).

Word Span. This test consists of repeating progressively longer word series (adapted from Christensen, 1975; Maruszewski, 1971).

Memory for Faces. In this test the child is given a pack of eight black-and-white photographs of children and is asked to sort them into two piles, one with girls and the other with boys. After that, eight pages are presented, each showing one of the previous photographs and two distractors. The child is to point out the photographs previously seen (adapted from Warrington & James, 1967).

Logical Learning. This test is performed as a continuation of the Storytelling test. Questions are asked about all details the child omitted in the free recall. The free-recall and cued-recall scores are added (cf. WMS, Christensen, 1975; Maruszewski, 1971).

Name Learning. Seven color photographs of children are presented three times. Each time the names of the children are presented once and rehearsed.

Delayed Recall. Half an hour after presenting the Memory for Faces test the child is asked to pick out the target photographs again among new distractors. Then he or she is asked questions on the content of the story in the Logical Learning test, as well as the names taught in the Name Learning test. The delayed-recall scores from the three tests are scored separately. Each test score is subtracted from the score of the corresponding test of immediate recall.

The Selective Auditory Attention test, The Sorting Test and Venger's Map Test are cognitively relatively demanding and should be discontinued if it is evident that the child does not comprehend the idea.

The complete assessment takes around two hours to present. In clinical practice the tests frequently are presented selectively, according to the child's problems.

Psychometric Characteristics

The test norms are expressed as *z*-scores, based on the means ($\bar{X}$) and standard deviations (SD) for each age group, and presented in tabular and graphic format (see Figure 4.2). The graphical norm figures show the test raw-score distributions of the various age groups in the form of "growth curves" with a line for the $\bar{X}$'s, surrounded by areas representing SD values +1, 0, −1, −2, and −3. A raw score is placed in the appropriate *z*-value area on the graph by referring to the precise age of the child on the horizontal axis.

Interscorer reliabilities range from 0.70 to 0.99, and measures of test homogeneity, calculated with the Kuder-Richardson formula (Ferguson, 1966), range from 0.59 to 0.89.

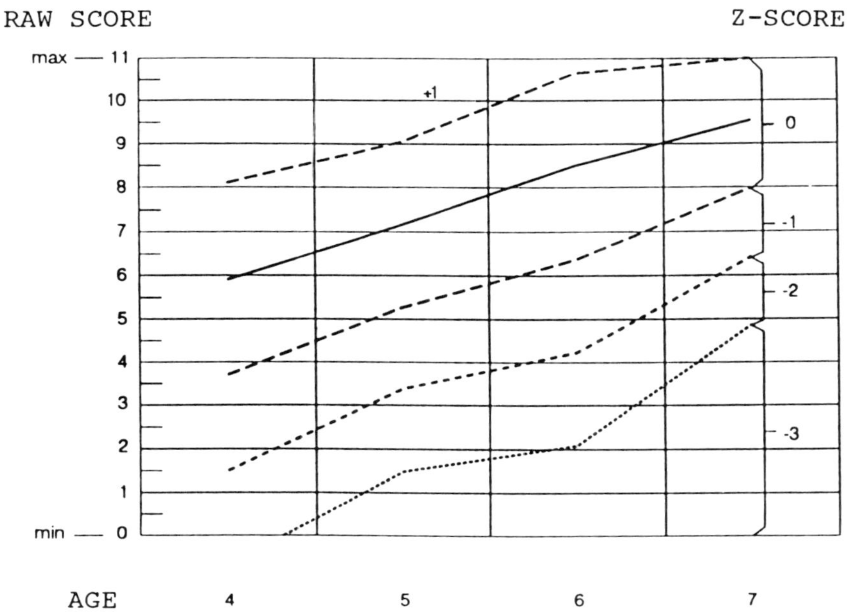

Fig. 4.2. Example of graphically presented test norm. A raw score is converted to a *z*-score by placing the raw score in the appropriate area on the graph, as determined by the child's precise age on the horizontal axis, and the raw score on the vertical axis. From Korkman (1990b). © 1990 Psykoiosi förlaget and Marit Korkman.

Test intercorrelations were calculated on the norm sample (N = 144 in Finnish version; N = 295 in Swedish version). The mean product-moment test intercorrelation coefficient for normal children was 0.26. After eliminating the effect of age, the mean partial intercorrelation was 0.11. In general, the language tests were more strongly intercorrelated than the tests belonging to other sections. The language tests also correlated with many of the tests from the other sections, indicating close relationship between language development and development of other areas. The whole set of intercorrelations is presented elswere (Korkman, 1988b).

A series of factor analyses was performed on the results of the Swedish norm sample. Because the tests were many compared to number of subjects, factor analyses were performed on the five parts of the NEPSY separately. The aim was to evaluate the homogeneity of the test sections and to eludicate the content of the tests. The Relative Concepts test and the MVPT were included across the factor analyses to clarify whether the factors obtained would be related to verbal or visual-spatial functioning. The factor analysis applied was an unrotated principal-components analysis.

In all five factor analyses, one main factor was seen in which most tests had loadings above 0.30. The Relative Concepts test and the MVPT also had high loadings in these factors. Only three of the tests described above did not have loadings above 0.30 on the main factor: a time score on the Visuo-Motor Precision test, a rotation score on the Block Construction test, and the Left-Right Orientation test (Korkman, 1990a). The results seem to indicate that cognitive development in normal children is relatively homogeneous. The same is not necessarily true for children with developmental disorders.

The clinical validity of the NEPSY has been evaluated in a series of studies of which three are reported below.

Clinical Application of the NEPSY

The NEPSY is amenable both to use as a fixed battery or as a process-oriented, hypothesis-driven device, or any intermediate approach (see Mattis, 1992; Tramontana & Hooper, 1988). Even applying individual tests from the NEPSY for some specific purpose is possible. In practice, however, the NEPSY has mostly been used in accordance with the traditions of process-oriented, hypothesis-driven assessment.

The NEPSY assessments are usually performed as the neuropsychological part in a multidisciplinary context. Other data on the child's complaint or the referral question, obstetric, developmental, and family history, school achievement, neuromotor evaluations, speech and language evaluations, evaluations by occupational therapists, and previous psychological evaluations are gathered collectively by the team. The accumulating data influence the assessment, the intervention, and the follow-up. Every child undergoes a program that is individually planned and tailored to suit his or her special needs and circumstances.

The content of the neuropsychological assessment depends on the cause of referral. The main causes may be grouped in these categories: (1) learning disorders or questions about development in some of the child's cognitive areas (e.g., development of language and speech); (2) suspicion or exclusion of brain dysfunction in connection with perinatal risks, behavior disorders, psychosomatic or somatic complaints or diseases, medical treatment that may affect CNS functions, intrauterine exposure to drugs, and so on; (3) clear evidence of brain dysfunction or damage, such as epilepsy, acute brain injury or disease, cerebral palsy, or hydrocephalus.

For learning or developmental problems and when brain dysfunction is to be excluded, the neuropsychological assessment may start with a core test battery consisting of the WPPSI or WISC-R, if not already performed, and some sensitive tests representing the main domains of neuropsychological functioning. In addition to the child's general intelligence, the WPPSI and the WISC-R yield data on whether a specific language problem (verbal IQ), a visual-spatial problem (Block Design and Object Assembly), or an arithmetic problem (Arithmetics) is present. Tests that are sensitive in discriminating children with learning disorders and brain dysfunction from normal control children, and also represent the main domains, are the Inhibition and Control test, the shortened form of the Token test, the Repetition of Words and Nonwords test, the Naming Tokens test, the VMI, the Visuomotor Precision test, and the Name Learning test (Korkman, 1988a, 1990b). From these preliminary core assessments, areas needing further investigation are specified.

In the more detailed part of the assessment, a stated problem is analyzed by separately assessing the components of the disturbed function. If the child presents with an attention problem, tests in the attention section are applied. If a poor result on the VMI is found, assessment with the sensory-motor and the visual-spatial tests may be needed. Frequently, the results of this second-level assessment may call for further analyses. If the tests in the language section indicate that the patient's primary problem is articulation, the assessment may be continued by also assessing the sensory-motor functions to delineate the motor problem more clearly.

Where brain pathology is clearly present, including epilepsy, brain tumor, or trauma, detailed examination is frequently desired to observe all aspects of the abnormality. Such a child may undergo a more comprehensive standard assessment, including the WPPSI or WISC-R, the complete NEPSY, and some complementary tests. Test that are almost always applied along with the NEPSY are the Token test, VMI, Grooved Peg Board (Kløve, 1964), and a dichotic listening technique (Korkman & Levänen, 1992).

The test results may be presented in a straightforward manner so as to describe a child's pattern of strengths and weaknesses. They may also be interpreted for primary and secondary deficiencies, in a manner comparable to Luria's principles of syndrome analysis. According to this principle, the components of disturbed functions are assessed separately to specify the weak link in the chain of subprocesses. A primary deficiency cannot usually be observed with one test, however, for every performance is complex and relies on several abilities. The primary deficiency underlying the cognitive disturbance has to be inferred by analyzing the pattern of findings. The inference is based on expectations of what would be the logical consequences of a hypothetical deficiency (Luria, 1970, 1973, 1980). If the test findings for a child referred for delayed speech or language development include normal verbal comprehension and naming, as well as fluent though poorly articulated speech, but instead oromotor and, eventually, manual precision problems, the primary deficiency seems to be speech articulation and oromotor coordination rather than a language disorder.

This type of interpretation relies heavily on the examiner's knowledge and views of the various learning disorders in children. For example, many authors see dyslexia as mainly a language problem (Bradley, 1989; Pennington, Van Orden, Smith, Green, & Haith, 1990; Scarborough, 1990; Vellutino & Scanlon, 1989), whereas other studies report a visual-motor or visual-spatial subtype of dyslexia (Korhonen, 1991; Spreen & Haaf, 1986). Adherents to these differing views may interpret a test profile that includes visual, verbal, and dyslexic deficiencies differently. The neuropsychological diagnosis is thus related to theory more than to specific tests.

If a test finding seems to indicate a deficiency such as poor auditory, phonemic analysis, this finding should be verified by applying at least one additional test of similar or closely related type (Wilson, 1992). Many of the NEPSY tests do tap closely related areas of functioning and may frequently verify each other. Many other tests may also be applied to verify findings obtained with the NEPSY. (For reviews of such additional tests, see Korkman, 1990a; Mattis, 1992; Spreen & Strauss, 1991; Wilson, 1992.)

Further, test findings and interpretations may also be validated against findings in everyday life. A finding of manual motor problems should have some practical correspondence or ecological validity in the form of poor handwriting, artwork, or handicraft.

A third source for verifying an interpretation is the internal consistency of the findings. The primary deficiency should be accompanied by secondary findings that are logical consequences of the former. An outspoken naming problem in the Color Naming test should be followed by difficulties also in the Token Test and the Naming Tokens test, because these tests too involve knowing the names of colors. Some problems are also likely to occur in other naming tests, specifically the Naming Body Parts and the Name Learning tests. This part of the interpretation thus takes the form of hypothesis testing. Keep in mind, however, that complex functions have considerable flexibility, and a deficiency in one subcomponent may be compensated for by strengths in others. Furthermore, normal development may vary not only interindividually, but also intraindividually, because the pace of development in different domains may be uneven. Some irregularities in the test patterns may therefore have to be tolerated.

Some times a brain dysfunction or damage can be localized by neuroimaging techniques or in brain surgery. These cases may provide opportunities to study anatomical and functional correlates. Especially in acute brain pathology or surgery, a follow-up is frequently conducted, which may provide an occasion to study the process of recovery.

Most children receive some type of remediation: physiotherapy, speech and language therapy, occupational therapy, neuropsychological habilitation, or special education. The neuropsychological findings are utilized to assist in planning these activities. The remediation also requires evaluating the outcome and a follow-up. Children may therefore have a long history of assessments and intervention. During this longitudinal treatment it is possible and desirable to provide at least one complete, standard assessment not only to children with trauma or epilepsy but also to children seen for learning disorders.

Illustrative Case

The NEPSY assessment is illustrated by a six-year-old girl. Anna was chosen because she had epilepsy (Epilepsia Focalis Generalisata), so that the complete NEPSY was performed, and because she was found to have a relatively frequent type of language disorder.

Anna was the third of five siblings. She and two of her siblings had mild delays in speech acquisition as well as articulation problems persisting until age five. Pregnancy and delivery were uneventful, except for placental calcification. Early development was normal. At age two years Anna began to have short episodes of stumbling and problems with balance. Some months later seizures appeared, with tonic extension of limbs and jerking eye movements. The EEG revealed generalizing spike slow wave bursts, starting in the left temporal area. Later, bursts seemed also to originate in the right hemisphere. The seizures responded well to medication and were subsequently reduced to one or two per year. On the neurological examination, status was normal, and an MRI examination was judged to be normal.

On the neuropsychological assessment Anna was cooperative and appeared well adjusted. She was not very talkative, but her speech seemed normal in fluency, articulation, prosody, and pragmatics. Intelligence, as measured by the WPPSI, was: verbal IQ = 95; nonverbal IQ = 96. The NEPSY test profile is presented in Figure 4.3.

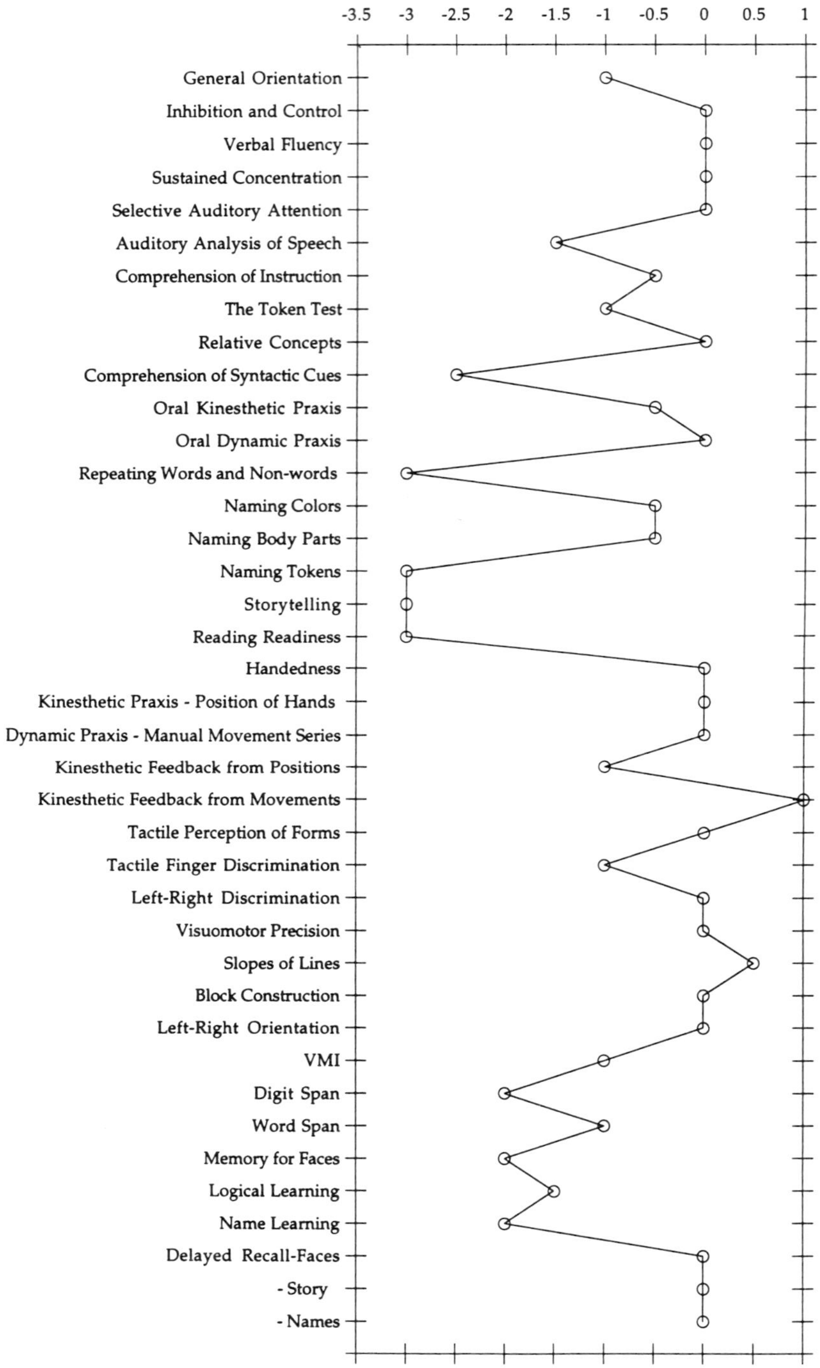

Fig. 4.3. Test profile of a six-year-old girl with epileptic seizures, EEG abnormalities originating in the left temporal area, and language disorder.

Preliminary inspection of the test profile revealed problems mainly in language and memory. The former findings were consistent with the history of a mild delay in speech and language development. Therefore, the language section in the NEPSY test profile was examined first to evaluate whether a language disorder was present. The analysis focused on presence or absence of problems in expression, articulation, receptive functions, and naming.

In expressive speech, Anna's performance on the Word Fluency test was normal. She failed the Storytelling test, but comparing this result to that of the cued recall of the story, the latter was also found to be very poor. The probable explanation was failure to comprehend and consequently to remember the relatively complex story. Because Anna's speech was fluent it was concluded that she did not have a primary expressive language disorder.

Her performances on the Repeating Words and Nonwords test was poor, indicating difficulty in repeating novel and phonemically complex words. The cause may be either oromotor problems or poor auditory, phonemic decoding of speech. Anna's speech development had earlier been characterized by poor articulation. But Anna did not have signs of oral dyspraxia on the Oral Kinesthetic Praxis and Oral Dynamic Praxis tests, and her speech was normal. Thus, it seemed Anna's difficulties in repeating complex words might be accounted for by an auditory, phonemic decoding impairment. Mild impairments were seen, however, on two manual kinesthetic and tactile perception tasks. These results could indicate a mild delay in sensory-motor differentiation, which may have contributed to Anna's earlier problems in articulation.

The receptive tests gave consistent findings of problems in decoding and reception, evident in the Auditory Analysis of Speech test, the Comprehension of Instructions test, the Token test, and the Comprehension of Syntactic Cues test. The decoding, receptive-language deficiency thus was an obvious primary problem that was sufficient to explain Anna's delay in speech and articulation development, failure to comprehend and remember complex narration, and failure to repeat unfamiliar and phonemically complex words.

Anna also performed poorly on the naming tests and the Name Learning test. Such results almost always accompany receptive problems, but they may also occur independently. The naming problems may thus be both primary and secondary.

Beyond the language problems, impairment appeared on the VMI. Such an impairment may be related to either perceptual or motor problems. Anna showed no other signs of perceptual problems, but her performances on the Kinestetic Feedback from Positions and the Tactile Finger Discrimination were mildly impaired. Consequently, poor ability to copy designs may have been related to a mild problem in sensory-motor differentiation, becoming apparent only on relatively complex and demanding tasks.

In memory, Anna had poor results throughout the tests of immediate recall. On the Delayed Recall test, she did not, however, show increased memory decay that would have confirmed global memory problems. Further, the poor result on the Memory for Faces task was not confirmed by a validation test, the visual memory test of the ITPA, or the visual and spatial perceptual NEPSY tests. The memory problem thus seemed to be restricted to verbal recall, and may have been secondary to the receptive language impairments.

The primary deficiencies of Anna thus seemed to be (1) poor phonemic analysis of speech and mild receptive language impairment, leading to secondary problems in name retrieval and verbal learning. It also explained the earlier delays in speech and articulation development; (2) naming problems that may be both secondary to the receptive problems and partly independent, primary problems; and (3) insignificant delay in sensory-motor differentiation, causing subtle graphomotor problems and contributing to the earlier articulation problems.

Comparing the findings to everyday performance, Anna had no difficulties understanding speech in everyday life. This finding is typical for children with mild receptive language disorder; their impairments frequently become apparent only on specialized tests and as learning problems in school. For Anna, reading and spelling problems were thus to be expected when she started school (in Finland, children start school at age seven). Subsequently, Anna has had severe problems in reading and spelling, and has been referred to a special class.

Anna also underwent a dichotic listening test and the Grooved Pegboard test. On the former she showed absence of a right-ear advantage, whereas, on the latter, fine-motor manual coordination was within normal limits, with an expected difference between the dominant right hand and the nondominant hand.

Now for the etiology. Anna's language disorder may be hereditary, for we found a clear familial history. On the other hand it could also be related to the seizures and caused by an underlying left-sided brain dysfunction. The mild sensory-motor impairment and absence of right-ear advantage did not support one etiological hypothesis more than the other, for they may occur in both etiologies, the former as an unspecific finding, and the latter as a sign of left-sided brain dysfunction. A possible hypothesis is that the two etiologies may be related. The occurrence of epilepsy in conjunction with hereditary language disorder is not typical, but children with developmental language disorders do have an increased frequency of EEG abnormality and epileptic seizures (Cheliout-Héraut, Picard, Turlan, Lacert, & De Lattre, 1992; Echenne, Cheminal, Rivier, Negre, Touchon, & Billiard, 1992). An explanation might be genetic predisposition to disturbance of neural migration, causing neural heterotopias, especially in the language regions of the brain (Geschwind & Galaburda, 1985).

Validation Studies

Three studies illustrate how NEPSY is used in research and provide validational data. The studies are previously published and are summarized here. The first provides evidence for the predictive validity of some of the NEPSY tests. The second study demonstrates the discriminative validity of the NEPSY. The third study demonstrates the application of the NEPSY in a follow-up study on treatment effects.

Predicting Attention Problems at School (Korkman & Peltomaa, 1991)

The aim in this study was to identify types of neuropsychological test profiles that could predict problems with attention in school. Kindergarten students at risk for attention problems were examined with NEPSY and their attention in school was predicted. At the end of the first school semester the children's attention was evaluated and the hit rate of the prediction was examined.

Subjects

A heterogeneous group of forty-six children with various test failures on school maturity assessments underwent neuropsychological assessments just before they started school.

The criteria for inclusion in the study were: (1) test failures of any type or degree in the school maturity assessments; (2) starting school in normal classes. Consistent with the criteria, the children showed signs of learning disorders but normal intelligence.

The ages were 6 years, 9 months to 7 years, 11 months. The mean WISC-R IQ was 105.7 (SD = 15.1).

Methods

The school maturity assessments were locally developed measures that included graphomotor tasks and tasks on visual-spatial perception, which also depended on attention.

The neuropsychological assessment included tests thought to be sensitive to disorders of attention and executive functions. These NEPSY tests were applied: General Orientation, Inhibition and Control, Sustained Concentration, Verbal Fluency, Comprehension of Instructions, and Venger's Map Test. Other tests selected as sensitive to disorders of attention and executive functions were: the Color Form test (Reitan-Indiana test battery), the Mazes test (WISC-R), the Coding test (WISC-R), the Matching Familiar Figures Test (MFFT; Kagan, 1966), the Square Test (Psykologien kustannus, 1986), and the Triangle Test (Psykologien

Table 4.1. Test Profiles of Preschool Children at Risk for Attention Problems in School.

Tests		Subgroups One ($n = 5$)	Two ($n = 16$)	Three ($n = 4$)	Four ($n = 7$)	Five ($n = 6$)	Total Group ($N = 46$)
General Orientation	$\bar{x}$ =	−1.7	−0.9	−1.0	−1.5	−1.0	−1.1
	sd =	0.8	1.2	0.9	0.7	0.9	1.0
Inhibition and Control	$\bar{x}$ =	0.5	−6.4	−0.7	−0.8	−5.0	−3.5
	sd =	1.2	3.1	1.1	1.6	10.0	4.7
Sustained Concentration	$\bar{x}$ =	−1.4	−2.6	−1.3	−1.6	−1.6	−1.9
	sd =	1.6	0.9	1.6	0.8	1.1	1.2
Comprehension of Instructions	$\bar{x}$ =	−5.3	−1.6	1.4	−2.5	−1.3	−1.8
	sd =	2.7	2.4	0.0	3.2	1.5	2.7
Verbal Fluency	$\bar{x}$ =	−1.0	−0.6	−0.4	−1.5	−0.2	−0.8
	sd =	0.4	0.9	1.1	0.5	0.8	0.9
Venger's Map Test	$\bar{x}$ =	−0.7	−1.4	−0.9	−0.6	−1.6	−1.1
	sd =	0.6	1.4	1.3	1.4	1.1	1.3
Color Form	$\bar{x}$ =	−1.2	−1.1	0.8	−4.3	−0.1	−1.6
	sd =	1.5	2.2	0.4	1.8	1.2	2.7
Mazes (WISC-R)	$\bar{x}$ =	3.6	1.4	4.0	−0.9	1.4	1.5
	sd =	2.0	2.1	0.9	1.8	2.9	2.4
Coding (WISC-R)	$\bar{x}$ =	−1.7	−0.8	−1.8	−1.6	−1.2	−1.2
	sd =	0.9	1.1	0.6	0.7	0.4	0.9
The Square Test	$\bar{x}$ =	−0.5	−0.7	−0.1	−1.0	−0.6	−0.7
	sd =	0.7	0.9	0.8	1.1	0.8	0.8
The Triangle Test	$\bar{x}$ =	0.2	−0.6	−0.7	−1.7	−1.2	−0.9
	sd =	0.9	0.9	0.9	0.3	0.5	0.9
MFFT, errors	$\bar{x}$ =	−0.2	−1.7	−0.6	−1.5	−4.0	−1.8
	sd =	0.8	1.1	1.0	1.1	1.3	1.5
MFFT, latencies	$\bar{x}$ =	−0.4	0.6	0.3	0.9	0.9	0.5
	sd =	0.7	1.0	0.9	0.5	0.5	0.8

Note: Subgroup scores $\geqslant -1.5$ are underlined
From Korkman and Peltomaa (1991), by permission of *Journal of Abnormal Child Psychology*, 19:451–467.

kustannus, 1986). The latter two are Finnish tests constructed to assess problem solving, strategy generation, and planning ability.

For evaluating attention in school, the Conners Teacher Rating Scale (CTRS; Goyette, Conners, & Ulrich, 1978) was used. An all-around evaluation also was obtained from the teachers, reporting on the child's general ability to attend to school work and instruction.

The test profiles were classified into subgroups with the aid of a Q-type factor analysis (Nunnally, 1967). This method is well suited for studies in which the number of subjects is small in relation to the number of tests. A rotated Varimax factorial design was used.

Results

In the Q-type factor analysis, a five-factor solution was chosen. The factor subgroups explained 87% of the variance. The test profiles of the subgroups and the total group are presented in Table 4.1.

To test the differences in test profiles a repeated-measures MANOVA (Tabachnick & Fidell, 1989) was performed. The interaction effect of groups and tests, which expresses the differences in test profiles, was $F(48, 75) = 3.17$ ($p = 0.014$).

As may be seen in Table 4.1, subgroups 2 and 5 had three test findings that consistently pointed to impaired attention: poor results on the Control and Inhibition test, the Sustained Concentration test, and the MFFT. Thus, the hypothesis was that the children in these subgroups would have more attention problems in school than those in the other subgroups.

Subgroup 4 also had some findings indicating attention problems, but because these impairments were relatively mild this subgroup was placed together with those in which attention problems were not likely to occur. Other test findings in this subgroup seemed to indicate problems with problem solving and strategy generation (see Table 4.1).

On follow-up, 15 (68.2%) of the 22 children in subgroups 2 and 5 were evaluated by the teachers to have attention problems. In contrast, only 5 (31.2%) of the 16 children in subgroups 1, 3, and 4 were evaluated as inattentive. The difference was tested with a Cohen's kappa (Cicchetti & Sparrow, 1981). The coefficient (0.41) expressed a fair hit rate.

The CTRS did not discriminate significantly between the collapsed subgroups, although subgroups 2 and 5 did have the highest ratings of inattention according to this measure as well.

Conclusions

Test profiles characterized by poor results on the Inhibition and Control test, the Sustained Concentration test, and the MFFT seemed to predict attention problems in school. These tests are intended to measure the ability to control impulses, persistence on cognitive tasks, and selective attention, respectively. One common factor in these findings could be poor ability to sustain a mental, cognitively defined set, which makes these children prone to distraction by irrelevant stimuli and competing impulses.

Test Profiles of Children with Attention Disorder and/or Specific Learning Disorder (Korkman & Pesonen, 1994)

This study compares the neuropsychological test profiles of children with attention deficit hyperactivity disorder (ADHD), specific learning disorder (LD), and children with both disorders (ADHD+LD).

Subjects

Sixty children were recruited from schools in Helsinki, Finland. The children were eight-year-old second-grade students in normal classes, 15 girls and 45 boys. These criteria were applied: the child should have (1) either ADHD or specific LD, according to the specified test scores, presented below; (2) average (≥90) verbal or performance IQ; and (3) no significant emotional or conduct problems. Selection included attention ratings performed by the class teachers, a spelling test given by special-education teachers, and intelligence testing and behavioral evaluations performed by school psychologists. Specific ADHD was found in 21 of the children, specific LD in 12, and ADHD + LD was found in 27 children.

Mean verbal IQ was 97.8 for the ADHD group, 89.2 for the LD group, and 90.6 for the ADHD+LD group. The corresponding performance IQ means were 102, 98.3, and 93.5, respectively. The groups did not differ in performance IQ, age, or gender, but they did differ in verbal IQ. This difference probably reflects a tendency toward language disorders of children with reading and spelling disorder. The difference was not eliminated because doing so would be likely to distort true differences between the groups.

Methods

The criterion measure in selecting children with ADHD consisted of a rating of attention and hyperkinesia based on the DSM-III criteria for ADD with hyperactivity (American Psychiatric Association, 1980). The criterion for ADHD was that the children should be evaluated to have attention deficit (4 or 5 points on a 5-point scale) on at least 7 of the 12 items. The criterion measure for identifying specific LD was a spelling test (Helsingin kouluvirasto, 1984), similar to the spelling test in the Wide Range Achievement test (Jastak & Wilkinson, 1984). The criterion for spelling problems was an error score ≥60% on the spelling test.

The label specific LD in this context refers to disorders observed in spelling only. Characteristics of the Finnish language (abundant vowels, phonetic spelling) make elementary reading relatively easy to acquire, whereas spelling causes more problems (abundant double vowels and consonants). In the lower grades the spelling test is therefore sensitive to dyslexic problems (Korkman & Pesonen, 1994).

The neuropsychological assessment included these NEPSY tests: Inhibition and Control, Selective Auditory Attention, Auditory Analysis of Speech, Relative Concepts, Storytelling, Naming Tokens, Handedness, Tactile Finger Discrimination, Visuomotor Precision, Digit Span, Name Learning, and Delayed Recall of Story. These complementary tests also were included: an overall evaluation of attention and ability to concentrate, performed by the schoolteacher, the Token test, VMI, MVPT, Block Design (WISC-R), and Object Assembly (WISC-R).

Results

The test profiles of the three groups are presented in Figure 4.4. Group differences were tested with ANOVA. Because of a tendency toward unequal distribution of gender, a two-way ANOVA (3×2) was applied, with gender as the second source of variation. As may be seen in Figure 4.4, significant differences appeared in the expected directions in 6 of the 19 tests. The effect of gender was not significant. The ADHD and the LD groups were also compared separately with t-test comparisons. Significant group differences appeared in four tests. The group differences were tested further by applying a repeated-measures ANOVA to the test profiles based on the seven discriminating tests (Tabachnick & Fidell, 1989). Comparing the three groups, the interaction ratio was $F(14, 399) = 3.75$ ($p = 0.02$). Comparing only the ADHD and the LD groups, the F-ratio was $F(7, 217) = 6.55$ ($p = 0.01$).

Conclusions

Children with specific ADHD had relatively good overall performance, but their performances on the Inhibition and Control test were significantly poorer than those of the LD group. Children with specific LD had significantly poorer test means on the Auditory Analysis of Speech test, the Digit Span test, and the Storytelling test. These results agreed with views of poor impulse control as one of the main characteristics of ADHD children (Barkley, 1988; Douglas, 1984; Korkman & Peltomaa, 1991). They also corresponded to the findings of linguistic and phonological awareness problems as major types of dysfunction underlying reading disorders (Bradley & Bryant, 1985; Vellutino & Scanlon, 1989; Wagner & Torgesen, 1987).

In spite of significant group differences, the results on the Auditory Analysis of Speech test were above zero even for the specific LD group, because the children were somewhat older than the oldest test norm group and they had received more reading and spelling education.

Children with ADHD+LD demonstrated the same deficiencies as both the ADHD and the specific LD groups. They were also impaired on the Selective Auditory Attention test and the evaluation of ability to concentrate, indicating even more pervasive attention problems than were evident in the ADHD group. Further, their performances on the Visuomotor Precision test and the VMI were poor, which may indicate a problem with motor precision as well.

Along with the differences between groups, the Name Learning test was impaired (≤ -1) in all groups. Naming Tokens was also relatively

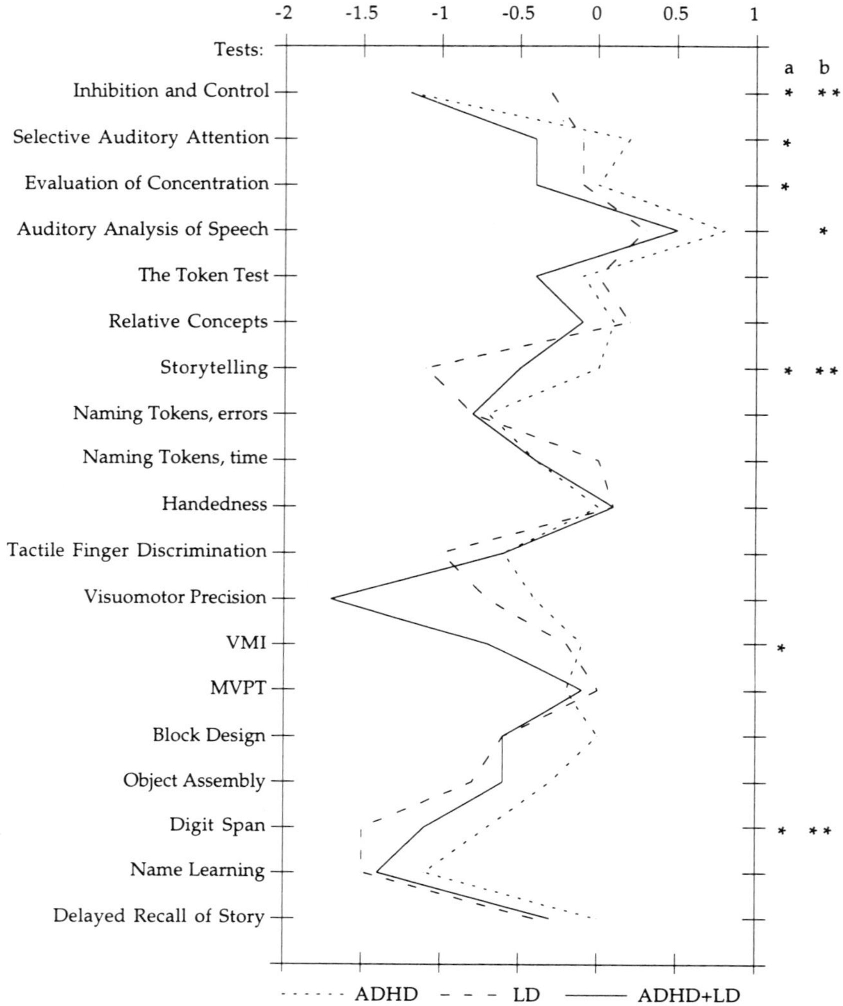

Fig. 4.4. Test profiles of children with ADHD (n = 21), specific LD (n = 12), and ADHD+LD (n = 27). Results show (a) significant differences among the ADHD, LD, and ADHD+LD groups, as compared by ANOVA (df = 2, 54); and (b) significant differences between ADHD and LD groups compared by t-test (df = 58). $^{a}p \leq 0.05$; $^{b}p \leq 0.01$. From Korkman and Personen (1994), *Journal of Learning Disabilites*, *27*, 383–392. Copyright 1994 by PRO-ED, Inc. Reprinted by permission.

poor for all groups. These findings seem to indicate that name retrieval is impaired not only in LD children but also in ADHD children, perhaps because of poor rehearsal strategies and active memorizing (Douglas & Benezra, 1990; Robins, 1992).

Preventive Treatment of Dyslexia in Children with Language Impairments (Korkman & Peltomaa, 1993)

This study investigated the efficiency of a treatment program developed to reduce the risk of reading and spelling problems in preschool children with language problems. The children were assessed before the treatment and one year after it had ended, at the end of their first school year.

Subjects

From a pool of 92 preschool children with developmental problems, 63 children were selected according to these criteria: (1) subnormal performances ($z = \leq -1$) on at least three of seven language tests; (2) intelligence within normal limits (IQ <85 on the WPPSI or <80 on the WISC-R). Of these children, 33 were assigned to experimental treatment. Seven of the children did not start school in normal classes and had to be excluded from follow-up, reducing the experimental group to 26 children, all males. A corresponding control group was formed of 20 male children who did not participate in the treatment.

The mean age of the experimental group was 6 years, 1 month and that of the control group 6 years, 2 months. The mean verbal IQ of the experimental group was 91.7 and the mean performance IQ was 96.0. The corresponding means for the control group were 92.3 and 96.7. The groups did not differ in age, intelligence, SES, or neuropsychological pretreatment findings.

Methods

The neuropsychological pre- and posttreatment assessments included these NEPSY tests: Inhibition and Control, Sustained Concentration, Selective Auditory Attention, Auditory Analysis of Speech, Relative Concepts, Naming Tokens, Storytelling, Tactile Finger Discrimination, Word Span, Name Learning, and Delayed Recall of Names. The Token test and the VMI were also included.

To evaluate reading and spelling skills, four tests were applied: one reading test of a word-attack type, two reading-comprehension tests, and one spelling test (Ekebom, Kivelä, & Härkönen, in press).

The treatment was performed in small groups (two to six children) with one 45-minute session weekly during the year before the children started school. The training included phonemic-awareness exercises and preliminary grapheme-phoneme conversions on a letter-sound or two-letter nonsense-syllable level. The latter type of exercise was meant to reduce difficulties in acquiring and retrieving phonemic labels for letters. Reading meaningful words was not taught, nor was writing or spelling (Peltomaa & Korkman, in press). In addition to the training, many children from both groups received speech therapy and most participated in kindergarten and preschool activities.

Table 4.2. Posttreatment Means (SD in parentheses) for Experimental Group ($n = 26$) and Control Group ($n = 20$) on Tests of Reading and Spelling.

Tests	Experimental group	Control group	t (df = 44)
Mechanical Reading	41.5 (14.6)	34.5 (19.2)	1.4 n.s.
Reading Comprehension 1	9.3 (1.9)	6.8 (3.7)	2.86**
Reading Comprehension 2	6.3 (2.2)	4.4 (3.2)	2.37*
Spelling	22.0 (5.0)	17.0 (9.6)	2.11*

*$p \leq 0.05$.
**$p \leq 0.01$.

Results

On the posttreatment needing and spelling tests, performed at the end of the first school year, the experimental group significantly outperformed the control group on three of the four measures (see Table 4.2).

On neuropsychological pretreatment assessments the groups did not differ significantly. On the posttreatment assessments, the experimental group outperformed the control group on the Relative Concepts test, $t(44) = 2.8$, $p < 0.01$, and on the Naming Tokens test, $t(44) = 2.9$, $p < 0.01$. When a Bonferroni correction was applied these differences were no longer significant.

On within-group comparisons the experimental group improved significantly on two attention tests (the Sustained Concentration and the Selective Auditory Attention tests) and two language tests (the Auditory Analysis of Speech and the Storytelling tests). The control group deteriorated on one measure, the VMI.

Conclusions

The results indicated that preschool training in phonemic awareness and grapheme-phoneme conversions may significantly reduce the risk of reading and spelling problems in school. The group differences on neuropsychological pre- and posttreatment measures did not reach significance, indicating that the training had the clearest effects on the target skills instead of being mediated by some change in underlying neuropsychological functions. The experimental group improved significantly, however, on the Sustained Concentration and the Selective Auditory Attention tests, and on the Auditory Analysis of Speech and the Storytelling tests, indicating improvement in both attention and linguistic performance. On the posttreatment assessments, the experimental group also outperformed the control group on the Relative Concepts test and the Naming Tokens test before a Bonferroni correction. Because the tests applied were so numerous, this correction may have deflated the results heavily. Thus, it seems possible that the capacity for name acquisition and retrieval may be crucial as prerequisites for reading and spelling. This possibility should be explored further in a larger study.

Discussion

A neuropsychological assessment instrument, NEPSY, was constructed to analyze cognitive and psychomotor disorders in four- to eight-year-old children. The NEPSY includes 38 tests from attention and executive functions, language, sensory-motor functions, visual-spatial functions, and learning and memory. The simultaneous standardization of the tests permits presenting the results in the form of test profiles.

The broad range of simultaneously standardized tests is the main characteristic and major benefit of the NEPSY. The breadth of tests allows for a comprehensive survey of neuropsychological functions. The assessment is still detailed enough, though, to permit thorough inspection of selected functional domains. The simultaneous standardization equalizes the tests, alleviating the difficulties of interpreting and drawing conclusions connected with tests that are standardized on different norm groups.

The NEPSY approach offers the benefits of employing a qualitative as well as a quantitative approach to neuropsychological assessment. The tests represent the main aspects of cognitive functions, permitting qualitative analysis of a stated disability. At the same time the tests are constructed as psychometric scales yielding quantitative measures of performances.

Another advantage of the NEPSY is its connection to a theoretical framework making it possible to interpret the results according to neuropsychological theory. In constructing the tests, one main objective was to utilize and integrate prevailing theoretical views and traditions of assessment. New tests were designed where theoretically motivated to cover some aspect of functioning. The basic theoretical view underlying selection of the tests was the view expressed most explicitly by Luria (1973, 1980) that complex cognitive and psychomotor functions are composed of separate components. The separate tests represent the components considered to be decisive for normal execution of important functions. Many theoretically motivated test ideas other than those of Luria were also adopted (e.g., Benton, Hamsher, Varney, & Spreen, 1983; Berg, 1948; Boehm, 1969, 1971; Manuilenko, 1975; Warringon & James, 1967).

The NEPSY was designed for relatively young children, for whom lack of neuropsychological instruments has been most evident. As demonstrated in the study of preventive treatment of dyslexia (Korkman & Peltomaa, 1993) the NEPSY is amenable to application as a basis for planning intervention, and for follow-up evaluations on the effects of intervention. The NEPSY may thus, it is hoped, enhance the possibilities for early intervention.

On the negative side the Finnish version was standardized on very few children. The size of the Swedish sample was more appropriate. Another shortcoming is the narrow range of ages—four to eight years. Although other tests are available for older children, a comprehensive package of simultaneously standardized neuropsychological tests is still lacking. Further, the narrow age range of the NEPSY provides for too limited follow-up. In the American version of the NEPSY (Korkman, Kirk, & Kemp, in press), these shortcomings are corrected. The age range is extended to three to twelve years, and the tests are standardized on an appropriate number of children from each age band.

The NEPSY was not designed to assess all aspects of neuropsychological functioning. Intelligence, asymmetries of function as measured by dichotic, tachistoscopic, and manual-dexterity techniques, and autistic disorders are not part of the NEPSY and need to be assessed by other measures. Another domain not included was assessment of social competence and perception and expression of emotions. Although it is increasingly recognized that learning disorders may occur specifically in this and related psychosocial domains, such disorders have been assessed most successfully when applying indirect, inferential, or observational techniques (Harnadek & Rourke, 1994; Rourke & Fuerst, 1992; Semrud-Clikeman & Hynd, 1990). Valid models for assessment with direct tests are still lacking.

The three studies reported in this context illustrate how the NEPSY is applied in subgroup studies, predictive studies (Korkman & Peltomaa, 1991), discriminative studies (Korkman & Pesonen, 1994), and treatment studies (Korkman & Peltomaa, 1993). The studies demonstrated about specific tests that poor performance on the Inhibition and Control and the Sustained Concentration tests predicted attention disorders in a group of preschool children. Second-grade pupils with ADHD also performed poorly on the former test. Tests that were specifically impaired in school-age LD children with dyslexic problems were the Auditory Analysis of Speech test, the Storytelling test, and the Digit Span test. The two former language tests also improved most in treating phonological awareness in preschool, language-disordered children. The Name Learning and Naming Tokens tests were impaired not only in LD children but also in ADHD children, indicating that these name-retrieval tests may be sensitive to both learning and attention disorders. Indirect evidence was obtained that children with pervasive ADHD were specifically impaired on the Selective Auditory Attention test. The case study indicated that performances on the verbal-learning tests may be secondarily impaired in language disorders. Further evidence on the validity of specific NEPSY tests is presented elsewhere (Korkman, 1988a, 1990b; Korkman & Häkkinen-Rihu, 1994). Validity has not yet been demonstrated for every test, however.

Finally, the NEPSY has some limitations in its theoretical underpinnings. The theoretical view underlying the instrument is generic and leaves open many specific questions. Interpreting a result therefore depends on the examiner's views, as pointed out earlier. One example could be interpreting poor verbal learning results, which may be considered secondary to problems with attention and strategy, to language disorders, or as primary problems themselves. Another example, mentioned above, is interpreting visual and spatial impairments in relation to dyslexia. Such open questions, however, are not specific to the NEPSY approach—rather, they are common to child neuropsychological theory in general, and are challenges for future research. It is hoped that the NEPSY will be a useful tool for such research and will enhance theoretical understanding of children's cognitive disorders.

References

Alahuhta, E. (1978). *BMA-testi. Testi puhe-, lukemis- ja kirjoittamishäiriöiden primaarioireiden kartoittamiseksi.* [The BMA test: A test for the clarification of the primary symptoms of disorders of speech, reading and spelling]. Report No. 292/1978. Jyväskylä University.

Alin-Åkerman, B., & Nordberg, L. (1980). *Griffiths utvecklingsskalor I och II.* [Griffiths' Developmental Scales I and II]. Stockholm: Psykologiförlaget.

American Psychiatric Association. (1980). *Diagnostic and Statistical Manual of Mental Disorders* (3rd ed.). Washington, DC: American Psychiatric Association.

Anastasi, A. (1982). *Psychological testing* (3rd ed.). New York: Macmillan.

Annett, M. (1970). A classification of hand preference by association analysis. *British Journal of Psychology, 63,* 343–358.

Auzias, M. (1975). *Enfants gauchers, enfants droitiers.* [Left-handed children, right-handed children.] Actualités pédagogiques et psychologiques. Paris: Delachaux et Niestlé.

Barkley, R.A. (1988). Attention. In M.G. Tramontana & S.R. Hooper (Eds.), *Assessment issues in child neuropsychology* (pp. 145–176). New York: Plenum Press.

Beery, K.E. (1983). *Visual-Motor Integration.* Monograph. Cleveland: Modern Curriculum Press.

Beery, K.E., & Buktenica, N.A. (1967). *Developmental Test of Visual-Motor Integration.* Cleveland: Modern Curriculum Press.

Benton, A.L., Varney, N.R., & Hamsher, K.deS. (1975). *Judgment of Line Orientation, form B.* Iowa City: University Hospitals.

Benton, A.L., Hamsher, K.deS., Varney, N.R., & Spreen, O. (1983). *Contributions to Neuropsychological Assessment*. New York: Oxford University Press.

Berg, E.A. (1948). A simple objective technique for measuring flexibility in thinking. *Journal of General Psychology, 39,* 15–22.

Boehm, A.E. (1969). *Boehm Test of Basic Concepts. A*. New York: Psychological Corporation.

Boehm, A.E. (1971). *Boehm Test of Basic Concepts. B*. New York: Psychological Corporation.

Borg, G. (1977). *Visual Gestalt Ability*. Stockholm: Psykologiförlaget.

Bradley, L. (1989). Predicting learning disabilities. In J.J. Dumont & H. Nakken (Eds.), *Learning Disabilities. Vol. 2. Cognitive, Social and Remedial Aspects* (pp. 1–17). Amsterdam: Swets & Zeitlinger.

Bradley, L., & Bryant, P. (1985). *Rhyme and Reason in Reading and Spelling*. International Academy for Research in Learning Disabilities Series. Michigan: University of Michigan Press.

Cheliout-Héraut, F., Picard, A., Turlan, D., Lacert, P., & De Lattre, J. (1992). Dysphasies et anomalies paroxystiques. *ANAE, 4,* 177–184.

Christensen, A.-L. (1975). *Luria's Neuropsychological Investigation*. Copenhagen: Munksgaard.

Christensen, A.-L. (1984). The Luria method of examination of the brain-impaired patient. In P.E. Logue & J.M. Schear (Eds.), *Clinical neuropsychology: A multidisciplinary approach* (pp. 5–28). Springfield, IL: Charles C. Thomas.

Cicchetti, D.V., & Sparrow, S.A. (1981). Developing criteria for establishing interrater reliability of specific items: Application to assessment of adaptive behavior. *American Journal of Mental Deficiency, 86,* 127–137.

Colarusso, R.P., & Hammill, D.D. (1972). *Motor-Free Visual Perception Test*. California: Academic Therapy Publications.

Cronbach, L.J. (1984). *Essentials of psychological testing* (4th ed.). New York: Harper & Row.

DeRenzi, E., & Faglioni, P. (1978). Normative data and screening power of a shortened version of the Token Test. *Cortex, 14,* 41–49.

DeRenzi, E., & Vignolo, L.A. (1962). The Token Test: A sensitive test to detect disturbances in aphasics. *Brain, 85,* 665–678.

Diller, L., Ben-Yishay, Y., Gerstman, L.J., Goodkin, R., Gordon, W., & Weinberg, J. (1974). *Studies in cognition and rehabilitation in hemiplegia* (Rehabilitation Monograph No. 50). New York: New York University Medical Center Institute of Rehabilitation Medicine.

Douglas, V.I. (1984). Attentional and cognitive problems. In M. Rutter (Ed.), *Developmental neuropsychiatry* (pp. 281–329). London: Churchill Livingstone.

Douglas, V.I., & Benezra, E. (1990). Supra-span verbal memory in attention deficit disorder with hyperactivity normal and reading disabled boys. *Journal of Abnormal Child Psychology*, *18*, 617–638.

Echenne, B., Cheminal, R., Rivier, F., Negre, C., Touchon, J., & Billiard, M. (1992). Epileptic encephalographic abnormalities and developmental dysphasias: A study of 32 patients. *Brain and Development, 14,* 216–225.

Ekebom, U.-M., Kievlä, A., & Härkönen, I. (in press). *Lukemisen ja kirjoittamsen screening-testi. Luokat 1 ja 2.* [Screening test of reading and spelling. Grades 1 and 2]. Helsinki: PJK Test House.

Ferguson, G.A. (1966). *Statistical analysis in psychology and education* (2nd ed.). New York: McGraw-Hill.

Frostig, M., Lefever, W., & Whittlesey, J.R.W. (1963). *The Marianne Frostig Developmental Test of Visual Perception. 1963 standardization*. Palo Alto, CA: Consulting Psychologists Press.

Geschwind, N., & Galaburda, A.M. (1985). Cerebral lateralization: Biological mechanisms, associations, and pathology. I. A hypothesis and a program for research. *Archives of Neurology, 42,* 428–459.

Golden, C.J. (1987). *Luria-Nebraska Neuropsychological Battery: Children's Revision*. Los Angeles: Western Psychological Society.

Goyette, C.H., Conners, C.K., & Ulrich, R.F. (1978). Normative data on revised Conners Parent and Teacher Rating Scale. *Journal of Abnormal Child Psychology, 2,* 221–236.

Harnadek, M.C.S., & Rourke, B.P. (in press). Principal identifying features of the syndrome of non-verbal learning disabilities in children. *Journal of Learning Disabilities*, *27*, 144–154.

Helsingin kouluvirasto (1984). *Ensiluokkalaisen luki-vaikeus*. [Dyslexia of the first-grade pupil]. Publications of Helsinki School Department, No. 6. Helsinki: Author.

Isaacs, B., & Kennie, A.T. (1973). The Set Test as an aid to the detection of dementia in old people. *British Journal of Psychiatry, 123,* 467–470.

Jastak, J.F., & Wilkinson, G.S. (1984). *The Wide Range Achievement Test-Revised*. Wilmington, DE: Jastak Associates.

Kagan, J. (1966). Reflection-impulsivity: The generality and dynamics of conceptual tempo. *Journal of Abnormal Psychology, 71,* 17–24.

Kløve, H. (1963). Clinical neuropsychology. In F.M. Forster (Ed.). *The medical clinics of North America, Vol. 47* (pp. 1647–1658). New York: Saunders.

Korhonen, T. (1991). An empirical subgrouping of Finnish learning-disabled children. *Journal of Clinical and Experimental Neuropsychology, 13,* 259–277.

Korkman, M. (1980). *NEPS—Lasten neuropsykologinen tutkimusmenetelmä*. [NEPS—A Neuropsychological assessment for children]. Helsinki: Psykologien Kustannus.

Korkman, M. (1988a). *NEPSU—Lasten neuropsykologinen tutkimus. Uudistettu versio*. [NEPSU—A neuropsychological investigation for children. Revised version]. Helsinki: Psykologien kustannus.

Korkman, M. (1988b). *NEPSY: A proposed neuropsychological test battery for young developmentally disabled children*. Doctoral dissertation. Helsinki University.

Korkman, M. (1988c). NEPSY: An adaptation of Luria's investigation for young children. *The Clinical Neuropsychologist, 2,* 375–392.

Korkman, M. (1990a). *NEPSY. Neuropsykologisk undersökning: 4–7 år. Svensk Version*. [NEPSY. Neuropsychological investigation: 4–7 years. Swedish version]. Stockholm: Psykologiförlaget.

Korkman, M. (1990b). The development of a neuropsychological investigation for children. In M. Hietanen, J. Vilkki, M.-L. Niemi, & M. Korkman (Eds.), *Clinical neuropsychology. Excursions into the field in Finland* (pp. 11–17). Helsinki: Suomen Psykologinen Seura.

Korkman, M., & Peltomaa, K. (1991). A pattern of test findings predicting attention problems at school. *Journal of Abnormal Child Psychology, 19,* 451–467.

Korkman, M., & Levänen, S. (1992). *Dikoottinen koe. Käsikirja* [The Dichotic Test. Manual]. Helsinki: PJK Test House.

Korkman, M., & Peltomaa, K. (1993). Preventive treatment of dyslexia by a preschool training program for children with language impairments. *Journal of Clinical Child Psychology, 22,* 277–287.

Korkman, M., & Häkkinen-Rihu, P. (1994). A new classification of developmental language disorders (DLD). *Brain and Language*, *47*, 96–116.

Korkman, M., Kirk, U., & Kemp, S.L. (in press). *NEPSY. Neuropsychological Assessment of Children*. San Antonio, TX: Psychological Corporation.

Korkman. M., & Pesonen, A.-E. (1994). Comparison of neuropsychological test profiles of children with attention disorders and/or learning disorder. *Journal of Learning Disabilities*, *27*, 383–392.

Kuusinen, J., & Blåfield, L. (1974). *Psykolingvististen kykyjen testi ITPA* [The Illinois test of psycholinguistic abilities]. Publications of the Institute of Pedagogical Research No. 234/1974. University of Jyväskylä.

Lezak, M.D. (1983). *Neuropsychological assessment* (2nd ed.). New York: Oxford University Press.

Luria, A.R. (1970). *Traumatic aphasia* (Trans. D. Boden). Paris: Mouton.

Luria, A.R. (1973). *The working brain*. London: Penguin Books.

Luria, A.R. (1980). *Higher cortical functions in man* (Trans. B. Haigh; 2nd ed.). New York: Basic Books.

Manuilenko, Z.V. (1975). The development of voluntary behavior in pre-school-age children. *Soviet Psychology, 4,* 65–115.

Maruszewski, M. (1971). Unpublished test material. Personal communication.

Mattis, S.M. (1992). Neuropsychological assessment of school-aged children. In F. Boller & J. Grafman (Eds.), *Handbook of neuropsychology, Vol. 6: Child neuropsychology* (pp. 395–415). Amsterdam: Elsevier.

McCarthy, D. (1972). *The McCarthy Scales of Children's Abilities*. New York: Psychological Corporation.

Nunnally, J.C. (1967). *Psychometric theory*. New York: McGraw-Hill.

Peltomaa, K., & Korkman, M. (in press). *Enhancing the Readiness to Acquire Reading and Spelling of Language-Disordered Children: A Preschool Treatment Program*. (M. Korkman, Trans.). Helsinki: PJK Test House.

Pennington, B.F. (1991). *Diagnosing learning disorders: A neuropsychological framework*. New York: Guilford Press.

Pennington, B.F., Van Orden, G.C., Smith, S.D., Green, P.A., & Haith, M.M. (1990). Phonological processing skills and deficits in adult dyslexics. *Child Development, 61,* 1753–1778.

Psykologien kustannus (1986). *Lasten hahmotustestisarja. Ohjeet. Kokeiluversio*. [Children's perceptual test series. Instructions. Experimental version.] Helsinki: Author.

Reitan, R.M. (1979). *Manual for administration of neuropsychological test batteries for adults and children*. Tucson, AZ: Reitan Neuropsychological Laboratories.

Rey, A. (1964). *L'Examen clinique en psychologie*. Paris: Presses Universitaires de France.

Robins, P.M. (1992). A comparison of behavioral and attentional functioning in children diagnosed as hyperactive or learning-disabled. *Journal of Abnormal Child Psychology, 20,* 65–82.

Rourke, B.P., Bakker, D.J., Fisk, J.L., & Strang, J.D. (1983). *Child neuropsychology: An introduction to theory, research and practice*. New York: Guilford Press.

Rourke, B.P., Fisk, J.L., & Strang, J.D. (1986). *Neuropsychological assessment of children: A treatment-oriented approach*. New York: Guilford Press.

Rourke, B.P., & Fuerst, D.R. (1992). Psychosocial dimensions of learning subtypes: Neuropsychological studies in the Windsor Laboratory. *School Psychology Review, 3,* 361–373.

Russell, E.W. (1986). The psychometric foundation of clinical neuropsychology. In S. Filskov & T.J. Boll (Eds.), *Handbook of clinical neuropsychology. Volume II* (pp. 45–80). New York: Wiley & Sons.

Scarborough, H.S. (1990). Very early language deficits in dyslexic children. *Child Development, 61,* 1728–1741.

Semrud-Clikeman, M., & Hynd, G.W. (1990). Right hemisphere dysfunction in nonverbal learning disabilities: Social, academic, and adaptive functioning in adults and children. *Psychological Bulletin, 107,* 196–209.

Spreen, O., & Benton, A.L. (1965). *Neurosensory Center Comprehensive Examination for Aphasia*. Victoria, BC: University of Victoria.

Spreen O., & Haaf, R.G. (1986). Empirically derived learning disability subtypes: Replication attempts and longitudinal patterns over 15 years. *Journal of Learning Disabilities, 19,* 170–180.

Spreen, O., & Strauss, E. (1991). *A compendium of neuropsychological tests: Administration, norms, and commentary*. New York: Oxford University Press.

Tabachnick, B.G., & Fidell, S.L. (1989). *Using multivariate statistics* (2nd ed.). New York: Harper & Row.

Terman, L.M., & Merrill, M.A. (1973). *Stanford-Binet Intelligence Scale*. Manual for the third revision, form L-M. Boston: Houghton Mifflin.

Tramontana, M.G., & Hooper, S.R. (1988). Child neuropsychological assessment: Overview of current status. In M.G. Tramontana & S.R. Hooper (Eds.), *Assessment issues in child neuropsychology* (pp. 3–32). New York: Plenum Press.

Vellutino, F.R., & Scanlon, D.M. (1989). Auditory information processing in poor and normal readers. In J.J. Dumont & H. Nakken (Eds.), *Learning Disabilities. Vol. 2. Cognitive, social and remedial aspects* (pp. 19–46). Amsterdam: Swets & Zeitlinger.

Venger, L.A., & Holmomsakya, V.V. (1978). *Diagnostika umst vennogo razvitja doskolnekov*. [Diagnosing the cognitive development of preschool children] Moscow: Pedagogika.

Vilkki, J., & Laitinen, L.V. (1974). Differential effects of left and right ventrolateral thalamotomy on receptive and expressive verbal performances and face-matching. *Neuropsychologica, 12,* 11–19.

Wagner, R.K., & Torgesen, J.K. (1987). The nature of phonological processing and its causal role in the acquisition of reading skills. *Psychological Bulletin, 101,* 192–212.

Warrington, E.K., & James, M. (1967). An experimental investigation of facial recognition in patients with unilateral cerebral lesions. *Cortex, 3,* 317–326.

Wechsler, D. (1977). *Wechslerin älykkyystestistö esikouluikäisille* [Wechsler Primary and Preschool Scale of Intelligence]. Helsinki: Psykologien kustannus.

Wechsler, D. (1984). *Wechsler Intelligence Scale for Children-Revised. Käsikirja* [Wechsler Intelligence Scale for Children-Revised. Manual]. Helsinki: Psykologien kustannus.

Wilson, B.C. (1992). The neuropsychological assessment of the preschool child: A branching model. In F. Boller & J. Grafman (Eds.), *Handbook of neuropsychology, Vol. 6: Child neuropsychology* (pp. 395–415). Amsterdam: Elsevier.

CHAPTER 5

Advances in Neuropsychological Constructs: Interpreting Factor Analytic Research from a Model of Working Memory

ANTONIA A. FORSTER and INGRID N. LECKLITER

In this chapter we survey advances in child neuropsychological assessment by focusing on the construct validity of three major instruments. One is the progenitor of child neuropsychological batteries, the Halstead-Reitan Neuropsychological Test Battery for Older Children (HRB-OC); one is new, the Wide-Range Assessment of Memory and Learning (WRAML); and one is recently revised, the Wechsler Intelligence Scale for Children-Third Edition (WISC-III). A model of working memory (Aaron & Joshi, 1992; Baddeley, 1992) provides a framework for this survey.

The elaboration of neuropsychological theory as it relates to memory is a critical advance in the field as a whole. Specifically, the model is shifting from one of *capacity* (short-term and long-term memory) to one of *process* (working memory and executive function) (Aaron & Joshi, 1992). This shift is reflected by the increasing number of publications on working memory and executive function in the child neuropsychology literature (e.g., Gnys & Willis, 1991; Swanson, 1987; Welsh, Pennington, & Groisser, 1991; Wielkiewicz, 1990). As this theoretical shift has been integrated into test construction and interpretation, several advances in child neuropsychological assessment have resulted: First, our understanding of how major assessment instruments (specifically, the WISC-III, the WRAML, and the HRB-OC) measure working memory and executive function is improving. Second, we are conceptualizing how these constructs are related to previously established constructs such as "Freedom from Distractibility" or "Verbal Processing." Third, we are making progress toward a unified theory of neuropsychological functions. We discuss the implications of these themes for assessment instruments used in child neuropsychology in the context formed by surveying the construct validity of three major assessment instruments.

Construct validity for the WISC-III, WRAML, and HRB-OC can be established by two complementary methods: factor analysis and clinical hypothesis testing. The first approach is based on statistical analyses and the second on clinical analyses similar to those of Lezak (1983), Luria (1980), and Rourke & Brown (1986). Because each method has shortcomings they should be used together to inform both clinical analyses and development of theory.

As a whole, research shows that the factor structures of the WISC-R, WISC-III, WRAML, and HRB-OC are equivocal. Consequently, the clinician cannot rely wholly on factor structure to interpret findings. Instead, clinicians also use hypothesis testing, interpreting factors when they apply to an individual patient's protocol (Leckliter, Matarazzo, & Silverstein, 1986), and interpreting subtests individually when necessary (Gioia, 1991; Sattler, 1988). Yet, to interpret individual subtests, even those of the Wechsler Scales (the best-researched instrument in psychology), we need further studies that refine each subtest's specificity and demonstrate their construct validity (Kamphaus, 1993). Fortunately, the field is progressing by statistically establishing clusters or networks of tests that appear to measure similar constructs. This analysis should facilitate hypothesis testing.

In this chapter, we (1) provide a synopsis of the process model of working memory; (2) review recent factor analytic studies of the WISC-III, WRAML, and HRB-OC and their implications for construct validity, particularly as they relate to working memory; and (3) suggest the neuropsychological operations that underlie subtests from these three instruments, viewing them as tasks that involve working memory and executive function.

Working Memory

In recent memory research, a tripartite model known as working memory has proven productive (Baddeley, 1992). The three components of working memory, according to this model, are a central executive or attentional controller, and two subsidiary systems, a phonological loop and a visuo-spatial sketch pad. Other subsidiary systems, such as the kinesthetic, proprioceptive, and olfactory, are likely to exist but are not yet integrated into a model of working memory. The tripartite model defines working memory as the system that concurrently stores and manipulates information, and coordinates resources. A critical feature in this approach is a shift away from the idea of *capacity*, or seeing memory solely as a holding area (e.g., for a specific number of digits), and toward the idea that working memory is an operational *process* (e.g., forming associations between novel and familiar material) (Aaron & Joshi, 1992).

The central executive's role in cognitive function is complex but as yet has no precise operational definition. Baddeley describes the central executive as coordinating information from the two subsidiary systems. Swanson (1987) suggests that the central executive performs metacognitive strategies. Welsh et al. (1991) propose that executive processes facilitate goal-oriented behavior by allowing for planning, maintaining set, controlling impulses, and organizing search for information. In other words, executive processes help in handling, retaining, and accessing information that enters the two subsidiary systems. Driscoll (1993) suggests a positive relationship between the ways and degrees to which information is processed and how information is encoded and retrieved.

The roles of the phonological loop and visuo-spatial sketch pad are better understood than those of the central executive (Baddeley, 1992). Of the two subsidiary systems, the phonological loop is understood better than the visuo-spatial system (Baddeley, 1992; Welsh, Pennington, & Groisser, 1991), probably because the latter is more complex. Baddeley suggests that it consists of separable visual and spatial processes. Basic perceptual information such as acoustic or visual input initially enters the sensory register, namely echoic or iconic memory for acoustic and visual information, respectively (Aaron & Joshi, 1992; Baddeley, 1992; Driscoll, 1993; Sheslow & Adams, 1990). Relevant information is then transferred to short-term memory. The central executive is likely to have a role in determining relevance. Although phonological short-term memory has limited capacity, acoustic information can be retained through strategies such as rehearsal and chunking, via an articulatory control process, like inner speech (Baddeley, 1992). The *speed* at which these operations are performed is a critical feature of phonological processing, in part determining *capacity*. Some of this information is then transferred to long-term memory via executive processes, where it is relatively permanent (Driscoll, 1993).

The complex process of working memory may be disrupted by deficits in either of the two subsidiary systems, or in the central executive. Whereas weaknesses in either of the two subsidiary systems yield fairly circumscribed effects (Baddeley, 1992), weaknesses in the central executive can cause more widespread and disruptive effects. In this situation, test results often are difficult to interpret. Consequently, precise analysis of the component processes of current memory tasks is lacking (Baddeley, 1992). Inasmuch as working memory is a complex, evolving model, it must be bootstrapped from experimental research and clinical findings. Thus, our current memory tasks are somewhat arbitrarily constructed. Ideally, as the model evolves and the field approaches a unified theory of neuropsychological processes, assessment tasks will be redesigned to reflect these processes. To this end we must understand the processes that current tasks incorporate. Factor analytic studies shed light on these processes and are surveyed below for the WISC-III, WRAML, and HRB-OC.

Survey of Factor Analytic Studies for the WISC-III, HRB-OC, and WRAML

Wechsler Intelligence Scale for Children-Third Edition (WISC-III)

The construct validity of the Wechsler scales has been extensively researched with factor analytic studies. The various Wechsler scales have been interpreted as one-, two-, and three-factor tests (Kaufman, 1990; Leckliter, Forster, Klonoff, & Knights, 1986). Factor I (Verbal Comprehension) and Factor II (Perceptual Organization) have been stable for the most part across all the Wechsler scales, for all age groups. Factor III, (traditionally known as "Freedom from Distractibility"), has a less stable history (Kaufman, 1990). In restandardizing the WISC-R, another subtest (Symbol Search) was added, ostensibly to strengthen Factor III. Instead of lessening the uncertainties connected with Factor III, however, adding Symbol Search has led to further controversy about the factor structure of the WISC-III, raising again the question: How many factors does a Wechsler scale really have? With the Symbol Search test added, factor analyses reported in the WISC-III manual were interpreted as defining four factors for the WISC-III: the familiar Verbal Comprehension and Perceptual Organization factors, the elusive Factor III or "Freedom from Distractibility" factor, now consisting only of Arithmetic and Digit Span, and a new fourth factor, named "Processing Speed," consisting of Coding and Symbol Search (Wechsler, 1991).

WISC-III Factor Structure

Factor loadings from the WISC-III manual (Wechsler, 1991) for the total standardization sample are presented in Table 5.1. The factor structure of the WISC-III resembles that of the WISC-R in having strong Verbal Comprehension and Perceptual Organization factors (Kamphaus, 1993; Kaufman, 1979; Wechsler, 1991). Although Kamphaus (1993) argued that

Table 5.1. WISC-III factor loadings for the total sample.

Subtest	Factor 1	Factor 2	Factor 3	Factor 4
Information	**0.72**	0.29	0.25	0.09
Similarities	**0.72**	0.29	0.23	0.09
Vocabulary	**0.79**	0.22	0.18	0.16
Comprehension	**0.65**	0.19	0.17	0.19
Picture Completion	0.38	**0.53**	0.10	0.08
Picture Arrangement	0.33	**0.37**	0.08	0.25
Block Design	0.29	**0.70**	0.24	0.17
Object Assembly	0.26	**0.70**	0.11	0.14
Mazes	0.06	**0.36**	0.11	0.12
Arithmetic	0.41	0.27	**0.73**	0.15
Digit Span	0.26	0.19	**0.34**	0.18
Coding	0.11	0.13	0.09	**0.79**
Symbol Search	0.20	0.35	0.19	**0.56**

Note: Bold type reflects subtests' highest loading.
Source: Adapted from Wechsler (1991), with permission from The Psychological Corporation © 1991.

the Perceptual Organization factor is less well supported because Picture Arrangement and Mazes have relatively weak loadings (0.37 and 0.36, respectively), it is equally plausible that these tasks depend on additional processes, thus accounting for their relatively lower loading on Factor II. For instance, Picture Arrangement also appears to include some Verbal Comprehension (0.33) and visuo-spatial Processing Speed (0.25). These processes have face validity for this subtest, and are part of clinical hypothesis testing when an individual's performance on Picture Arrangement is interpreted.

Factor III is substantially weaker than it was on the WISC-R, both because it has lost Coding (0.09), and also because Digit Span's loading on Factor III is moderate (0.34) and does not exceed by a great deal its loading on Factor I (0.26). Factor IV is somewhat more robust in its loadings (Coding, 0.79; Symbol Search, 0.56).

Some disagree about the factor structure as presented in the WISC-III manual. Kamphaus (1993) finds that the first two factors remain interpretable, but raises serious questions about the interpretability of Factors III and IV. He advises against interpreting Factor III as distractibility, and suggests that the fourth factor be considered supplementary (i.e., interpreted only in the context of compelling case data). Pointing out the substantial loading of Arithmetic on Factor I (0.41), he suggests that clinicians should expect to see this score align with Factor I subtests a significant portion of the time (Kamphaus, 1993); Picture Arrangement and Digit Span may also fail to align with their factors, in accordance with their relatively low loadings (Kamphaus, 1993). He advises that only experienced clinicians interpret Factors III and IV and preferably after validity studies supporting these factors are available (Kamphaus, 1993).

Sattler (1992), in reanalyzing the standardization data, performs a maximum-likelihood factor analysis on the standardization group for the total sample and for *each* age group. He comments that the factor analytic results presented in the WISC-III manual were inconsistent among the total sample and the *four* age-group subsamples that were analyzed (ages 6–7, 8–10, 11–13, and 14–16 years). Consequently, he argues that analyzing by individual age groups rather than clustered age groups is more accurate. Because Factor III or "Freedom from Distractibility" did not appear for all four age groups, Sattler concludes that the four-factor model is "inappropriate," and argues for a three-factor solution that omits Factor III, and omits Picture Arrangement from Factor II (Sattler, 1992, p. 1046).

Roid, Prifitera, and Weiss (1993), in a study intended to replicate the WISC-III factor structure in an independent sample, argue that the eigenvalue rule that Sattler uses to define factors can result in inaccuracy, and that groupings across a wider age range improve the stability of factor loadings. These authors cite results from studies of small clinical samples, presented in the WISC-III manual (Wechsler, 1991), as criterion-related evidence that the four-factor solution is valid. Finally, Roid et al. (1993) argue that the Coding subtest had its lowest loading (0.09) on the WISC-III Factor III, and is therefore more accurately placed along with Symbol Search on Factor IV.

Historically, the two important questions about the factor structure of the Wechsler scales are: (1) How many factors do they really have? and, (2) What do the factors really mean? These two questions are addressed for the WISC-III in the next sections.

How Many Factors Does the WISC-III Really Have?

The number of factors obtained for the Wechsler scales has greatly depended on the types of groups studied (e.g., clinical versus normal standardization sample), age groupings (e.g., across all ages versus grouped by annual increments), and on the factor analytic methodology used (Kaufman, 1990; Leckliter, Matarazzo, & Silverstein, 1986). For example, a case can be made for considering the WAIS-R a one-, two-, or three-factor test (Kaufman, 1990). Experts do not agree which factor analytic methodology is appropriate under what circumstances; as a result, no one study or group of studies is likely to yield a definitive solution. Instead, factor structures vary across samples of individuals with different ages, clinical characteristics, and ability profiles, compared to samples homogeneous for these characteristics. Instead of being considered a problem, these differences across study samples should be used to elucidate processing differences across clinical or demographically diverse groups. For instance, age-based differences in WISC-III factor structure might contribute to a developmental model of neuropsychological processes.

Based on these premises, the true factor structure of the Wechsler scales is best resolved at the level of the individual test protocol (Kaufman, 1990; Leckliter, Matarazzo, & Silverstein, 1986). The decision on which factors to interpret is based on the clinical utility of particular factors for a specific individual. For example, for the WAIS-R, a three-factor solution provides the clinician with more hypotheses to test, and thus is preferable when it is appropriate (Leckliter, Matarazzo, & Silverstein, 1986). The decision to interpret a factor depends on whether the individual performed differently on tests comprising that factor than on tests comprising the other two (Kaufman, 1990).

By creating a fourth factor, adding Symbol Search to the WISC-III provides the clinician with more hypotheses to test. Further factor analytic studies are needed, using homogeneous clinical samples grouped according to age, to clarify unique factor solutions for the WISC-III with different groups of children at different ages. Although the factor structure of the WISC-III is a powerful interpretive tool (Kamphaus, 1993), the pattern of subtest loading does not conform to the factor structure for all children. Clinicians must therefore rely on a hypothesis-testing approach, integrate the results of groups of subtests, and perform a profile analysis (Rourke & Brown, 1986) to make sense of the child's cognitive abilities. In such cases it is mandatory to have other test results with which to combine WISC-III data, as well as school records and behavioral and personality information. Here the factor analytic approach to construct validity of entire tests gives way to that of individual subtests; this topic is taken up in a later section. Next we review the factor structure of the WISC-III, and its predecessor, the WISC-R, from the standpoint of what we may learn about working memory.

What Do the WISC-III Factors Mean?

At least as important as the issue of the real factor structure of the WISC-III is the issue of what the WISC-III factors mean. A very large literature covers the occurrence and interpretation of low scores on WISC-R Factor III among widely varied clinical populations. Wielkiewicz (1990) reviews studies on the meaning of low WISC-R Factor III scores, and lists associated findings and possible hypotheses for low scores (see Table 5.2).

The range of problems that co-occur with low Factor III scores demonstrates that poor performance on Factor III is not confined to one diagnostic group, however broadly one defines it. Neither does one processing deficit account for poor performance on Factor III. The name "Freedom from Distractibility" is therefore misleading, for interpretation of low Factor III scores may reflect problems other than distractibility.

Table 5.2. Associated findings and possible hypotheses for low scores on the WISC-R Third Factor.

Presence of a learning disability
Motivational problems in school
Poor reading ability, with weak short-term memory and visual motor integration
Low school achievement
Low arithmetic achievement
Difficulty in concentration or focusing attention
Poor sequential processing, related to difficulty in decoding
Poor executive problem-solving strategies (e.g., difficulty in shifting set)
Poor performance on trail making test, Part B
Somatic complaints
Residual attention deficit
Referral for evaluation of learning or behavior problems
Poor study skills
Distractibility
Deficits in motor development
Speech and language delays or disorders
Male

Source: Adapted from Wielkiewicz (1990), p. 94, with permission from the author.

Instead the WISC-R Factor III, and the WISC-III Factors III and IV, may be assessing children's use of working memory (Wielkiewicz, 1990). For example, subtests that comprise Factor III on the WISC-III (Arithmetic and Digit Span) may require use of the phonological loop more than the other subtests. Similarly, subtests that comprise Factor IV (Coding and Symbol Search) may require use of the visuo-spatial sketch pad to perform them accurately and quickly. Both factors are likely also to require an element of executive function, a topic addressed below. This reconceptualization of WISC-III Factors III and IV seems to be supported by the loadings of other subtests on these factors. Namely, Information, primarily a verbal memory task, loads moderately on Factor III; and Picture Arrangement, a task with many visual-processing demands, loads moderately on Factor IV. One might test whether Factor III reflects a phonological loop with executive requirements by determining how well Digits Backward loads on the factor. Presumably, Digits Backward would load higher than Digit Span as a whole because verbal rehearsal (inner speech) is one strategy commonly used to perform this task and, like Arithmetic, Digits Backward requires more mental operation (possibly executive function) than Digits Forward. Digits Forward merely requires verbal recapitulation with little need for complex mental operation. Digits Backward also might load more highly on Factor IV than Digits Forward, for some subjects use a visual-imaging strategy to hold the digits in memory. In summary, Factors III and IV may reflect aspects of working memory, with primary emphasis on the phonological loop and visuo-spatial sketch pad, respectively.

The Central Executive

Tasks requiring working memory are complex in that they tax the central executive and at least one of the two subsidiary systems. Executive skills are themselves complex and varied, and the nature of the executive component differs across tasks. One factor on which all Wechsler subtests load, "G," may reflect aspects of executive function or the "power" to perform multiple mental operations simultaneously, while holding information in storage, particularly when learning new information or problem solving in novel situations. Executive function may also, however, reflect ability to perform operations rapidly, while holding information in storage, called "flexibility" or "speed." Thus, tasks such as Arithmetic and Digits Backward emphasize the "power" aspect of executive function (performing arithmetic or transpositional operations while remembering numbers or number sequences). Coding and Symbol Search, on the other hand, form a factor that emphasizes the "speed" aspect of executive function (rapid visual scanning and writing, sequenced smoothly; holding some material in storage is helpful, particularly on Coding).

Evidence for such a multifactorial interpretation of the central executive comes from a factor analytic study of tasks currently used to assess executive function in children. Welsh et al. (1991) found that their battery of tasks formed three factors reflecting speeded responding, set maintenance, and planning. Their First Factor, labeled Fluid Speeded Response, is like the new WISC-III Factor IV in both name and skills assessed. Like Coding and Symbol Search, the tasks comprising the Fluid and Speeded Response Factor require visual planning, speeded response, and behavioral sequencing.

Subtest Interpretation

Understanding the psychometric relationships among the subtests, and between subtests and factors, aids in clinical interpretation. To take advantage of the power available in the network of skills these tests represent, however, one must be able to interpret the meaning of scores on individual subtests, and on combinations of subtests. This interpretive strategy is used by many clinicians and is commonly known as profile analysis (Rourke & Brown, 1986), yet little research has been aimed at the construct validity of individual WISC-III or WISC-R subtests, and little research has been aimed at the validity of profile analysis for individual protocols (Matarazzo, 1990). The factor analytic approach to construct validity seeks to cluster tasks that require similar skills to clarify what is being assessed. Ultimately, to understand the meaning of the aggregates, we need to understand the individual subtests and their subcomponents (Kamphaus, 1993).

Consequently, the clinician will find it useful to think about the WISC-III subtests in terms of the operations required for successful performance, especially for Factor III and IV subtests. To this end, Table 5.3 operationally describes each of these tasks. Instead of describing the tasks by listing nouns naming purported constructs measured by the subtests, as is normally given in texts that describe such instruments (e.g., Kamphaus, 1993; Kaufman, 1979; Sattler, 1992), Table 5.3 lists verbs describing the operations required for success on the Factor III and IV subtests. This shift is consistent with the growing view of memory as a process. Picture Arrangement is included because of its moderate loading on Factor IV. Table 5.3 is intended to help generate hypotheses; interpretations based on subtest scores or groups of scores are less reliable and valid than those based on IQ scores, and need correspondingly more supportive data from other sources before being offered in a report (Kamphaus, 1993).

In each of these tasks simultaneous demands are made on at least one subsidiary system and on the central executive. Each task combines these two major processes of working memory in a slightly different way, however. In Table 5.4, Factor III and IV subtests, and Picture Arrangement, are grouped according to the operations they share. For example, the task Digits Forward typically demands use of the phonological loop. Digits Backward also requires the phonological loop, although some individuals use verbal rehearsal via inner speech and others transfer the

Table 5.3. WISC-III Third and Fourth Factor Subtests: Operations required for successful performance.

Arithmetic	Holding verbally poresented information in short-term memory Discriminating relevant from irrelevant verbal information Retrieving number facts from long-term memory Performing basic numeric operations Understanding mathematical concepts (e.g., subtraction) Understanding orally presented arithmetic problems Verbal response
Digit Span *Forward*:	Attending to orally presented number sequences Holding and rehearsing orally presented numbers in phonological loop Repeating precise number sequences
Backward:	Attending to orally presented number sequences Holding and rehearsing orally presented numbers in phonological loop and/or transforming, holding, and rehearsing orally presented information in visuo-spatial sketch pad Manipulating and resequencing material held in short-term memory Understanding the spatial concept "backward" Verbal response
Coding	Discriminating among unfamiliar symbols Rapid visual scanning and matching Rapid shifting from one symbol to the next Holding unfamiliar symbols in visuo-spatial sketch pad Rapid copying of unfamiliar symbol, motor output Rapid sequencing of behaviors (scan, find, hold, write, shift) Holding arbitrary symbol–number pairs in visuo-spatial sketch pad
Symbol Search	Perceiving identity/differences among unfamiliar symbols Rapid visual scanning and matching Holding unfamiliar symbol in visuo-spatial sketch pad Rapid shifting from one symbol array to the next Rapid sequencing of behaviors (search, compare, decide, mark, shift) Motor output
Picture	Rapid visual scanning
Arrangement	Perceiving critical differences in visually depicted situations Interpreting social situations Inferring cause and effect Sequential processing, planning, and executing a logical sequence Motor output

verbal input to the visuo-spatial sketch pad (by visualizing the numerals). Unlike Digits Forward, Digits Backward requires ability to understand the spatial concept "backward" and manipulate the remembered numbers. This set of skills may be part of the central executive.

WISC-III Summary

The construct validity of the Wechsler factors III and IV is not crisp for good reason: these tasks as a group assess working memory, which

Table 5.4. WISC-III Third and Fourth Factor Subtests: Neuropsychological Constructs and Operations.

Global construct	Basic operation	Subtests
Sequential operations	Following a prescribed sequence of scanning, memory, and writing behaviors	Coding Symbol Search
	Creating a logical sequence of story segments	Picture Arrangement
	Remembering number sequences	Digit Span
Short-term memory	For precise number sequences	Digits Forward Digits Backward
	For arithmetic problems presented orally	Arithmetic
	For unfamiliar symbols	Coding (Symbol Search)
Information processing	Performing mental operations involving numbers	Arithmetic Digits Backward
Visual operations	Detecting critical visual detail	Picture Arrangement
	Rapid Visual Scanning	Coding Symbol Search (Picture Arrangement)
Motor operations	Rapid writing of symbols or marks	Coding Symbol Search
Auditory operations	Accurate encoding of auditory material	Arithmetic Digit Span
Logical operations	Arithmetic reasoning	Arithmetic
	Behavioral/social reasoning	Picture Arrangement
Executive operations	Rapid shifting to next stimulus	Coding
	Integrating related visual scenes	Symbol Search Picture Arrangement

comprises both short-term memory and executive skills. Other Wechsler subtests may assess executive skills with minimal emphasis on a memory component (e.g., Block Design, Object Assembly) (Wielkiewicz, 1990), or long-term memory with minimal emphasis on an executive component (Information). Factor subtests III and IV confound both of these dimensions of working memory (executive skills and holding information in storage), and thus may not form consistent factors in some samples and in many individual protocols. Consequently, the clinician may find interpreting an individual protocol more productive by considering the third and fourth factor subtests, and to a lesser extent Picture Arrangement, as a network that assesses components of working memory.

Although Factors III and IV of the WISC-III represent a somewhat better-articulated assessment of working memory than did the WISC-R Factor, III, many possible explanations remain for poor performance on either or both of these factors. Deficits in any one of the many skills listed in Table 5.3 can cause low scores. Because the WISC-III is not intended to be a complete neuropsychological battery, successful hypothesis testing requires additional measures. One of the Wechsler scales and the HRB-OC often have been used together for this purpose. The survey turns now to summarize factor analytic studies with the HRB-OC.

Halstead-Reitan Neuropsychological Test Battery for Older Children (HRB-OC)

The HRB-OC adds significant information beyond that provided by the Wechsler scales. For example, the WISC-R and the HRB-OC reportedly share only 10% of their variability (D'Amato, Gray, & Dean, 1988a). The variance that is unique to the HRB-OC also is clinically useful. Strom et al. (1987) reported that academic achievement scores for learning-disabled children were more accurately predicted (an increase of 16% to 30%) when the HRB-OC tests were added to WISC-R results. Rattan et al. (1989) investigated the association between the WISC-R factor structure and HRB-OC performance in a group of learning-disordered children. They reported that the HRB-OC predicted only 21% of the variance in WISC-R Factor III, 20.9% of the variance in WISC-R Factor II (Perceptual Organization), and 7.3% of the variance in WISC-R Factor I (Verbal Comprehension). These results indicate that the HRB-OC is not a redundant part of a battery including the Wechsler scales, and that HRB-OC test results are related more to performance, working memory, or executive function than they are to verbal comprehension skills.

Some understanding of the constructs measured by the HRB-OC can be gained by examining the factor analytic studies of the HRB-OC completed in the last few years. Table 5.5 summarizes the studies, HRB-OC measures they included, number and type of subjects, subject ages, and number of HRB-OC factors extracted. Table 5.5 makes clear, as stated by Batchelor et al. (1991), that understanding the constructs measured by the HRB-OC and understanding its psychometric properties in general, has been impeded by the lack of uniformity in HRB-OC tests administered across laboratories. Of the studies listed, only one (Batchelor, Sowles, Dean, & Fischer, 1991) included all the WISC-R variables and the standard HRB-OC measures whose scores are amenable to factor analysis. Only one study (Gatten, Krug, Brooks, Davis, & Dean, unpublished manuscript) included all the standard HRB-OC tests, exclusive of the Wechsler and other scales.

Besides problems of disparate test batteries across laboratories, several other difficulties impede clear interpretation of factor analytic studies on the HRB-OC. Only one study used normal children (Klonoff, 1971); the remaining studies used heterogeneous samples of referred or learning-disabled children. This variability complicates interpreting the studies' results because variation in composition of samples differentially influences factor structure. Using standard versus raw scores is another problem. Batchelor et al. (1991) and Gatten et al. (unpublished manuscript) transformed HRB-OC scores to standard scores using normative data provided in Knights & Norwood (1980). And yet, Knights & Norwood (1980) did not use standard instrumentation and instructions for the HRB-OC, and some of their samples were very small (Leckliter, Forster, Klonoff, & Knights, 1992). The extent to which these slightly different procedures and instruments might affect the derivation of standard scores is unknown. The remaining studies used raw scores, the traditional scoring procedure for HRB-OC variables. Using raw scores in factor analyses when scores from other instruments are in standard form may also be a problem. D'Amato et al. (1988b) hypothesized that the factor structure they obtained was affected by including raw scores.

Another potential problem with these factor analytic studies is that significant gender differences have been found in HRB-OC test performance among learning-disabled children, with males' scores superior to females' scores on many measures (Batchelor & Dean, 1990). Still, the studies listed in Table 5.5 included a heavy preponderance of males, and factor analyses were conducted on total samples instead of gender-segregated samples.

In spite of methodological problems, tentative conclusions based on these HRB-OC factor analytic studies have the potential to advance our knowledge in child neuropsychology. Among the strengths of these studies is that sample sizes in the LD and referred groups are appropriately large. Also, in most, a Wechsler scale, generally considered an essential concurrent measure, was included. A large factor analytic study of normal children using the HRB-OC and the WISC-R or WISC-III would have been ideal, but such a standardization, using nonreferred children, is a very costly multisite undertaking.

Table 5.6 summarizes the factors and their tests reported in the studies listed in Table 5.5. It excludes factors that did not include HRB-OC tests, however.

It is evident from Table 5.6 that several relatively consistent factors occur across studies. Table 5.7 lists the factors that were judged stable and all the tests that may load on them.

A factor was judged stable if tests loaded on it uniquely (i.e., nowhere else in the table), and if the constellation of tests comprising the factor occurred in at least three of the studies listed. In spite of evidence showing that Seashore Rhythm and Speech Sounds, as measures of auditory discrimination, are related to learning-disabled children's WISC-R subtest performance (Strom, Gray, Dean, & Fischer, 1987). Seashore Rhythm and Speech Sounds Perception did not consistently load on a specific factor across studies. Trail Making Test (TMT) Parts A & B also

Table 5.5. Factor analytic studies of the HRB-OC.

Study	Measures	*N*	Sample type	Age groups	# Extracted factors
Batchelor et al. (1991)	WISC-R	1,236	LD	9–10	6
				11–12	7
				13–14	7
	Category			All ages	7
	TPT				
	Speech Sounds				
	Seashore Rhythm				
	Trails A & B				
	Tapping				
	Grip Strength				
	WRAT Reading				
	WRAT Spelling				
	WRAT Arithmetic				
D'Amato, Gray, & Dean (1988a)	WISC-R	1,181	Learning Problems	8–16	6
	Category				
	TPT				
	Speech Sounds				
	Seashore Rhythm				
	Trails A & B				
	Tapping				
D'Amato, Gray, & Dean (1988b)	WISC-R	934	Learning Problems	8–16	7
	Category				
	TPT Times				
	TPT Memory				
	TPT Location				
	Trails A & B				
	Speech Sounds				
	Seashore Rhythm				
	WRAT Reading				
	WRAT Spelling				
	WRAT Arithmetic				
	PPVT				
Francis, Fletcher, Rourke, & York (1992)	Object Assembly	722	Referred	9–12	5
	Block Design				
	Picture Completion				
	Coding				
	Verbal IQ				
	Performance IQ				
	Full-Scale IQ				
	Trails A				

Table 5.5. *Continued*

Study	Measures	*N*	Sample type	Age groups	# Extracted factors
	Tapping Grip Strength Target Test Holes Mazes Grooved Pegboard				
Gatten et al. (unpublished)	Category TPT Speech Sounds Seashore Rhythm Trails A & B Tapping Grip Strength	800	LD	9–14	4
Kelly et al. (1992)	Category	652	LD	9–14	3
Klonoff (1971)	WISC (all) Category TPT Speech Sounds Trails A & B Tapping Matching Figures Matching Vs Star Concentric Squares Progressive Figures Color Form Target Test Marching Test Benton Sound Recognition Right-Left Orientation Reitan-Klove Lateral Dominance Klove Maze Coordination Grooved Steadiness Steadiness Grooved Pegboard Foot Tapping	200	normal	9–15	19

Table 5.6. HRB-OC factors across studies.

Batchelor et al. (1991)	Francis et al. (1992)	Gatten et al. (unpublished)	D'Amato, Gray, & Dean (1988a)[b]	D'Amato, Gray, & Dean (1988b)[b]	Klonoff 1971
1. Simple Motor Ability	1. Simple Motor Ability	1. Speed of Operation	2. Motor Speed & Strength	4. Developmental	7. Motor Speed
Grip Strength Tapping	Grip Strength Tapping	Grip Strength Tapping Category Seashore Rhythm	Tapping Category Seashore Rhythm Speech Sounds	Tapping Category Seashore Rhythm	Tapping
2. Verbal Comprehension			1. Verbal Comprehension	1. Verbal Comprehension	2. Verbal Fluency
Information Comprehension Similarities Vocabulary			Information Comprehension Similarities Vocabulary	Information Comprehension Similarities Vocabulary Arithmetic	Information Comprehension Similarities Vocabulary Arithmetic
3. Symbolic Languge Integration				2. School Achievement	
WRAT Reading WRAT Spelling WRAT Arithmetic Speech Sounds				WRAT Reading WRAT Spelling WRAT Arithmetic Speech Sounds (Trails B) (Arithmetic)	
4. Spatial Organization & Integration		2. Tactile Motor Integration	5. Spatial Speed of Operations	5. Spatial Speed of Operations	5. Tactile Discrimination Speed
TPT Times		TPT Times	TPT Times Trails A Trails B (Picture Arrangement)	TPT Times Trails A Trails B	TPT Times
					15. Alternation Between Conceptual Realms
					Trails A Trails B Picture Arrangement

5. Visual Organization[a]	2. Complex Visual-Spatial Relations		3. Perceptual Organization	3. Perceptual Organization	17. Analytic Synthetic Visual Motor Ability
Picture Completion	Picture Completion		Picture Completion	Picture Completion	
Block Design	Block Design		Block Design	Block Design	Block Design
Object Assembly	Object Assembly		Object Assembly	Object Assembly	Object Assembly
			Picture Arrangement	Picture Arrangement	
Category	TPT Total				Category
6. Spatial Memory[a]		4. Visuo-Spatial Memory	6. Spatial Memory	6. Spatial Memory	14. Tactile Retention
TPT Memory	—	TPT Memory	TPT Memory	TPT Memory	TPT Memory
TPT Location	—	TPT Location	TPT Location	TPT Location	TPT Location
			(Trails A)		
7. Complex Visually Guided Motor Activities	5. Speeded Motor Sequencing				
Coding	Coding				
Trails A	Trails A				
Trails B					
	Mazes				
		4. Attention	4. Attention/Processing Speed		
		Trails A	(Trails A)	(Trails A)	
		Trails B	(Trails B)		
		Category			
		Speech Sounds	Speech Sounds		
		Seashore Rhythm	Seashore Rhythm		
		Arithmetic	Arithmetic		
		Digit Span	Digit Span		
		Coding	Coding		

[a] Among the 9–10-year-olds were Factors 5 and 6 subsumed in Factor 2. Among the 11- to 14-year-old group Factors 5 and 6 were unique.
[b] HRB-OC scores in this study were not transformed to standard scores.
Tests listed in parentheses loaded higher on another factor.
Factor numbers reflect their order from the study in which they were derived.

Table 5.7. Stable HRB-OC factors.

Factor name	HRB-OC tests
Motor Speed/Strength	Grip Strength
	Tapping
Spatial/Tactile Speed	TPT Times
Spatial Memory	TPT Memory
	TPT Location

failed to load in a consistent pattern, appearing in two studies with Tactile Performance Test (TPT) timed scores, in one with Finger Tapping, in one with Tactual Performance Test Memory and Location, and in the remainder with WISC-R Factor III tests.

Similarly, the Category Test did not load consistently on a specific factor. In some studies it appeared with Grip Strength and Finger Tapping, in another study with WISC-R Performance subtests, and in yet another with Trail Making Test: Parts A and B, Speech Sounds, and Seashore Rhythm. Factor analysis of the Category Test by Kelly et al. (1992) might explain some of this variability. They found evidence for three factors in Category Test performance: Visuo-perceptual/Spatial Orientation, Visuo-Abstract Reasoning/Memory, Number Counting/Attention. This factor composition may account for the associations among the Category Test and WISC-R Performance tests that require visuo-spatial skills; and Trail Making Test: Parts A & B, Speech Sounds, and Seashore Rhythm tests that require visuo-spatial, attention/tracking skills, and flexibility. It is also possible that the lack of factor stability for the Category Test may be related to idiosyncratic factors such as design characteristics (e.g., item difficulty) that interact with subjects' response biases (Bertram, Abeles, & Snyder, 1990).

The Category Test has been described as measuring skills subserved by all areas of the cerebral cortex (Bertram, Abeles, & Snyder, 1990). It has also been described as evaluating the capacity to learn by a trial-and-error approach, to test hypotheses, and to correctly generalize a set once it proves successful. Poor performance may predict one or all of these: set maintenance in spite of failure, learning inefficiency, and memory problems (Reeder & Boll, 1992). These skills generally are deemed to fall in the realm of executive function and most neuropsychologists agree that, in adults, the Category Test makes demands on executive function and frontal activity. Nevertheless, Berg et al. (1984) hypothesize that the children's version of the Category Test does not measure frontal-lobe functioning in children as it does in adults. This hypothesis makes sense because the frontal lobes form connections to other brain areas throughout childhood (Thatcher, 1991), and are not fully myelinated in human beings until adolescence (Lehr, 1990). And yet, Category Test for children may tap executive processes without calling upon frontal functioning.

This notion is supported by research with nonhuman primates (Goldman-Rakic, Isseroff, Schwartz, & Bugbee, 1983). Grossly simplified, this research demonstrated that skills requiring intact prefrontal functioning among adult primates could be performed by juveniles despite damage or thermal deactivation (cryogenic depression) of the prefrontal area. Thus, although the Category Test may require complex executive functions across the life span, the areas that subsume these functions may change as the child matures to adulthood. This developmental process may further confound interpreting factor analytic studies of the HRB-OC that grouped all subjects into one mixed-age sample.

HRB-OC Summary

Factor analytic studies of the HRB-OC have many problems that confound clear interpretation of a factor structure. Disparate test batteries across labs, use of standardized and raw scores for analyses, collapse of scores across all age groups, predominance of clinical groups, and gender effects are some of the problems. Nevertheless, three factors seem to appear consistently across studies: motor speed/strength, spatial-tactile speed, and spatial memory. As yet, it is not clear how these factors relate to working memory. Several HRB-OC tests clustered inconsistently with different tests across studies. These tests seem related to executive functions, the biological substrate of which may change as the child matures. The likelihood that executive functions encompass a broad array of processes may account for some of the inconsistency in HRB-OC factor structure.

Wide-Range Assessment of Memory and Learning (WRAML)

Despite all the research focused on the Wechsler scales and Halstead-Reitan batteries, many neuropsychologists have found these instruments lacking in a comprehensive assessment of memory. The Wide-Range Assessment of Memory and Learning was developed recently to address this shortcoming in child neuropsychology. Research with this new instrument may further our understanding of executive processes and working memory.

The WRAML is the first comprehensive, well-standardized battery for assessing memory function in children ages 5 through 17 years. From the perspective in this chapter, it can be seen as assessing the two subsidiary systems of working memory. Although it was not intended to assess metamemory, executive process, or metacognitive strategies (Sheslow & Adams, 1990), the fact that working memory requires direction by the central executive (Baddeley, 1992) suggests that the WRAML subtests may reflect central executive processes to some degree.

The nine subtests comprising the WRAML were divided by the authors into three scales: Verbal Memory scale, Visual Memory scale, and Learn-

Table 5.8. WRAML scales and subtests.

Verbal Memory Scale	Assesses verbal rote memory on three tasks that increase in semantic complexity.
Number/Letter	Child repeats numbers and letters verbally presented.
Sentence Memory	Child repeats sentences of increasing length.
Story Memory	Child recalls two brief stories.
Visual Memory Scale	Assesses visual memory along a dimension of increasing meaningfulness.
Finger Windows	Child reproduces spatial sequences by pointing to holes in a card.
Design Memory	Child is asked to draw geometric designs remembered after a 10-second delay.
Picture Memory	Child is shown a complex, meaningful scene, followed by a similar scene, and identifies changes in the second picture.
Learning Scale	All subtests consist of four trials, and a fifth delayed trial. One verbal, one visual, and one cross-modal task comprise this scale.
Verbal Learning	Adapted from Rey (1958). Child repeats a list of words presented orally four times.
Visual Learning	Child recalls location of colored geometric designs over four trials, and a fifth delayed trial.
Sound-Symbol	Child learns to associate sounds and abstract figures, and to recall the sounds when the pictures are presented.

Source: Adapted from Sheslow & Adams (1990), pp. 11–12, with the authors' permission.

ing scale. Because the WRAML is a relatively new, and perhaps unfamiliar instrument, Table 5.8 summarizes its nine subtests.

These nine subtests provide a means for assessing memory across developmental stages and along several dimensions or constructs; namely, visual and verbal processes, recall and recognition, immediate and delayed memory, episodic and semantic memory, and single- or multiple-trial learning. The extent to which a child must organize or process information may also be considered.

As a measure of memory function, the face validity of the WRAML is high. Surprisingly, although correlations among WRAML subtests are all in the expected direction, they are lower than one would expect from subtest intercorrelations of other multidimensional scales such as the WISC-R and WISC-III. Number/Letter and Sentence Memory correlate best, in both the younger and the older groups (r = 0.59, 8 years and younger; r = 0.60, 9 years and older). Nearly all other WRAML subtest intercorrelations are below r = 0.30, and many are below r = 0.20. WRAML subtests appear to have high individual variance, extensively measuring unique processes (Gioia, 1991). Gioia argues that the WRAML factor structure reported in the manual failed to account for this high specificity among subtests. Accordingly, he reanalyzed the WRAML standardization data with a more conservative approach—namely, a

Table 5.9. Four-factor solutions for principal-factor analyses of WRAML standardization data, grouped by age.

	Factor 1		Factor 2		Factor 3		Factor 4	
Age in years	5–8	9–17	5–8	9–17	5–8	9–17	5–8	9–17
Subtests								
Picture Memory	0.24	**0.43**	0.03	0.08	0.08	0.20	**0.37**	0.20
Design Memory	**0.42**	**0.74**	0.11	0.10	0.06	0.10	**0.43**	0.19
Verbal Learning	0.22	0.26	0.14	0.18	0.27	0.26	**0.42**	**0.34**
Story Memory	0.09	0.23	0.23	0.20	0.16	**0.68**	**0.60**	0.25
Finger Windows	**0.38**	0.23	0.22	0.28	0.02	0.11	0.19	0.26
Sound Symbol	0.13	0.19	0.12	0.25	**0.58**	0.23	0.18	0.50
Sentence Memory	0.10	0.11	**0.93**	**0.74**	0.15	0.33	0.26	0.14
Visual Learning	**0.54**	**0.40**	0.12	0.11	0.23	0.13	0.14	**0.48**
Number/Letter	0.21	0.07	**0.58**	0.77	0.10	0.03	0.08	0.18

Source: Adapted from Gioia (1991), with the author's permission.

Principal Factor Analysis. His reanalysis failed to support grouping the nine subtests into three scales as presented in the manual (i.e., Verbal Memory, Visual Memory, Learning Index). Instead, he suggested that the WRAML factor structure varies with age. Data from his four-factor solutions are presented in Table 5.9.

Table 5.9 shows only one consistent factor across ages, specifically Factor II, composed of the Sentence Memory and Number/Letter subtests. This factor may reflect the phonological loop of working memory and may correspond, to some extent, to Factor III of the WISC-III. Nevertheless, because these two WRAML tests merely require precise recapitulation of orally presented verbal information, they are likely to require less executive processing than Digits Backward or Arithmetic. Accordingly, one might hypothesize that a factor analysis of WISC-III and WRAML standardization data, combined, might force Arithmetic back into a Verbal Comprehension factor, but Digit Span, particularly Digits Forward, Sentence Memory, and Number/Letter might cluster in a purer factor reflecting the phonological loop of working memory. As yet, such combined factor analyses have not been published.

Table 5.9 also shows some commonality across age in Factor I: Design Memory and Visual Learning seem to cluster on this factor. That Finger Windows and Picture Memory load uniquely on this factor for the younger and older groups, respectively, suggests that the factor may reflect a visual-spatial dimension. Perhaps this factor incorporates the visuo-spatial sketch pad of working memory. Speculatively, a factor analysis of combined WISC-III, WRAML standardization data might cluster Design Memory and Visual Learning with Coding and Symbol Search. Among younger children, Picture Arrangement and Finger Windows might join this cluster, or might form a separate cluster, for both tasks require a unique executive process, namely, sequential organization of visually input information.

Factors III and IV in Table 5.9 are more difficult to interpret from the perspective of working memory. That Sound-Symbol falls out as a separate factor for younger children, though, may not be so difficult to understand when one considers the similarity between this WRAML subtest and the initial process of learning to read. Both require the young child, usually between ages 5 and 8, to associate a written symbol (grapheme) with an oral sound (phoneme). This associative process, which is more novel for the younger than for the older child, requires the child to attend to critical visual features of the grapheme and pair them with acoustic features of the phoneme. Novel tasks require more processing by the central executive than familiar tasks. Consequently, for younger children, the WRAML Factor III may reflect a developmentally unique, critical period, in which they must use executive skills to form associations between symbols held in the two subsidiary systems of working memory (the phonological loop and visuo-spatial sketch pad), an unfamiliar task that becomes more automatic after reading is mastered.

Older children, particularly those who are good readers, may use different cognitive skills to perform the Sound-Symbol subtest. Interestingly, Sound-Symbol loads on WRAML Factor IV for older children. The three subtests that load on this factor (Verbal Learning, Visual Learning, and Sound-Symbol) have multiple-trial learning as one commonality. Thus, the effective use of rehearsal and the development of effective strategies to aid encoding and retrieval may be the cognitive constructs that underlie Factor IV for older children. Encoding and retrieval may be faster and more accurate when the operation to be performed or the information to be encoded is familiar. Consequently, although ability to rehearse and develop effective strategies for learning may reflect executive processes at all ages, the operations actually executed by the central executive are likely to differ among different age groups.

WRAML Summary

The WRAML is a new instrument that shows promise in both research and clinical contexts. Because it is still so new, however, additional research is needed. Preliminary factor analyses show that age is associated with the WRAML factor structure, and only one factor, rote verbal repetition, holds across ages. Factor analysis of the WISC-III and WRAML standardization data, combined and stratified across several age groups, might help explain this finding and elucidate a theory of developmental neuropsychology. For instance, does the WRAML Factor III, among five- to eight-year-olds, reflect a critical period in which the child uses executive processes that enable him or her to learn visual symbol–sound associations? Once these associations are learned, or automatized, do the executive processes called upon differ? The difference in factor loading of Sound-Symbol across different ages seems to affirm that they do. Ultimately, answers to these and related questions may help us better understand the processes involved in executive function, how these relate to the two subsidiary systems of working memory, and how these processes change as the child matures.

Conclusion

The tripartite model of working memory, which includes an executive control function and two subsidiary systems, the phonological loop and visuo-spatial sketch pad, provides a new way to organize the constructs that underlie the most commonly used child neuropsychological measures, the WISC-III, HRB-OC, and WRAML. Subtests that compose these instruments appear to differ in the demands they place on working memory. The new WISC-III Factors III and IV may reflect subtests that require a moderate to high degree of working memory, with Factor III (Arithmetic and Digit Span) primarily incorporating the phonological loop and Factor IV (Coding and Symbol Search) the visuo-spatial sketch pad.

A combined factor analysis of the WISC-III and WRAML subtests should cluster WISC-III subtests that demand working memory and WRAML subtests. For example, across ages 5 to 17 years, the WRAML Factor II subtests (Sentence Memory, Number/Letter) and WISC-III Factor III subtests (Arithmetic and Digit Span) should load on one factor because both appear to require working memory that incorporates the phonological loop. How WRAML Factor I subtests (Design Memory and Visual Learning for ages 5 to 17, Finger Windows for ages 5 to 8, and Picture Memory for ages 9 to 17) would cluster with WISC-III subtests is less clear hypothetically because of apparent differences in WRAML Factor I structure across ages. Some subtests would be likely to cluster with WISC-III Factor II subtests (Perceptual Organization) and others with WISC-III Factor IV subtests (working memory with visuo-spatial sketch pad). It is premature to offer reasoned hypotheses about clusters of WISC-III subtests and WRAML Factor I subtests until more is understood about how age or development influences the factor structure of child neuropsychological instruments.

In this vein, a child's age and level of development are associated with another important dimension to consider, namely familiarity versus novelty. The WISC-III subtests that load on Factors I and II may place fewer demands on working memory because many of them reflect knowledge or operations that become more familiar and practiced as the child matures (i.e., Information, Vocabulary, Comprehension, Picture Completion, Object Assembly, Mazes) or because they do not require that information be held in storage (i.e., Block Design, Mazes). Because the WRAML was designed to tap memory processes it would be expected to correlate just moderately with the Wechsler scale: most WRAML subtests probably place more demands on working memory than do most Wechsler scale subtests. Nevertheless, as proposed for the WISC-III subtests, the degree to which WRAML subtests require working memory may also vary in familiarity versus novelty. For example, among children ages 5 to 8, who are less practiced in associating graphemes and phonemes than older children, the WRAML Sound Symbol subtest may demand more of working memory than among older children, ages 9 to 17 years.

Factor analytic research with the HRB-OC further confirms that age and developmental level are important considerations for understanding a model of working memory and how it might organize our thoughts about the processes that underlie child neuropsychological tests. For example, Batchelor et al. (1991) report that two factors (Visual Organization and Spatial Memory) were unique among older children (ages 11 to 14) but were subsumed into a larger factor (Verbal Comprehension) among younger children (ages 9 to 10). D'Amato et al. (1988b) argue for a unique Developmental Factor that includes Finger Tapping, Category, and Seashore Rhythm Tests. Expanding knowledge about neurodevelopmental changes and age should inform how the field refines a model of working memory and how it relates to the processes that underlie child neuropsychological tests.

Advances in child neuropsychology occur as we better understand how our tests cluster and in which ways they are unique. The tripartite model of working memory can provide a skeletal structure on which to begin organizing some of these findings. Knowing the shortcomings in past research (e.g., disparate batteries and test standards across laboratories, using raw and standardized scores together in one factor analysis, collapsing across groups with disparate critical characteristics such as age or clinical versus normal status) should help inform future research design and reduce the confounds that interfere with clear interpretation of research results. Ultimately these advances, informed by advances in neurodevelopment and information processing, will allow us to bootstrap a theory of developmental neuropsychology and to refine our instruments.

References

Aaron, P.G., & Joshi, R.M. (1992). *Reading problems: Consultation and remediation*. New York: Guilford Press.

Baddeley, A. (1992). Working memory. *Science, 255,* 556–559.

Batchelor, E.S., & Dean, R.S. (1990). Sex differences in neuropsychological performance for children with reading deficits. *International Journal of Neuroscience, 50,* 95–102.

Batchelor, E., Sowles, G., Dean, R.S., & Fischer, W. (1991). *Journal of Psychoeducational Assessment, 9,* 16–31.

Berg, R.A., Bolter, J.F., Ch'ien, L.T., Williams, S.J., Lancaster, W., & Cummins, J. (1984). Comparative diagnostic accuracy of the Halstead-Reitan and Luria-Nebraska Neuropsychological Adult and Children Batteries. *International Journal of Clinical Neuropsychology, 6,* 200–204.

Bertram, K.W., Abeles, N., & Snyder, P.J. (1990). The role of learning and performance on Halstead's Category Test. *The Clinical Neuropsychologist, 4,* 244–252.

D'Amato, R.C., Gray, J.W., & Dean, R.S. (1988a). A comparison between intelligence and neuropsychological functioning. *Journal of School Psychology, 26,* 283–292.

D'Amato, R.C., Gray, J.W., & Dean, R.S. (1988b). Construct validity of the PPVT with neuropsychology, intellectual, and achievement measures. *Journal of Clinical Psychology, 44,* 934–939.

Driscoll, M.S. (1993). *Lateralization of short-term and long-term verbal and visuospatial memory functions in older and younger children with traumatic brain injury*. Unpublished doctoral dissertation, Pennsylvania State University.

Francis, D.J., Fletcher, J.M., & Rourke, B.P. (1988). Discriminant validity of lateral sensory motor tests in children. *Journal of Clinical and Experimental Neuropsychology, 10,* 779–799.

Francis, D.J., Fletcher, J.M., Rourke, B.P., & York, N.J. (1992). A five-factor model for motor, psychomotor, and visuo-spatial tests used in the neuropsychological assessment of children. *Journal of Clinical and Experimental Neuropsychology, 14,* 625–637.

Gatten, S.L., Krug, D., Brooks, D.A., Davis, B., & Dean, R.S. *Factor analysis of the Halstead-Reitan Neuropsychological Battery for Older Children*. Unpublished manuscript, Neuropsychology Laboratory, Ball State University, Indiana.

Gioia, G.A. (1991). *Re-analysis of the factor structure of the Wide Range Assessment of Memory and Learning: Implications for clinical interpretation*. Paper presented at the Nineteenth Annual Meeting of the International Neuropsychological Society, February 14, 1991, San Antonio, TX.

Gnys, J.A., & Willis, W.G. (1991). Validation of executive function tasks with young children. *Developmental Neuropsychology, 7,* 487–501.

Goldman-Rakic, P.S., Isseroff, A., Schwartz, M.L., & Bugbee, N.M. (1983). The neurobiology of cognitive development. In M.M. Haith & J.J. Campos (Eds.), *Handbook of Child Psychology* (Vol. II). *Infancy and Developmental Psychobiology* (pp. 281–344). New York: John Wiley and Sons.

Kamphaus, R.W. (1993). *Clinical assessment of children's intelligence: A handbook for professional practice*. Boston: Allyn & Bacon.

Kaufman, A.S. (1979). *Intelligent testing with the WISC-R*. New York: Wiley-Interscience.

Kaufman, A.S. (1990). *Assessing adolescent and adult intelligence*. Boston: Allyn & Bacon.

Kelly, M.D., Kundert, D.K., & Dean, R.S. (1992). Factor analysis and matrix in variance of the HRNB-C Category Test. *Archives of Clinical Neuropsychology, 7,* 415–418.

Klonoff, H. (1971). Factor analysis for neuropsychological battery for children aged 9 to 15. *Perceptual and Motor Skills, 32,* 603–616.

Knights, R.M., & Norwood, J.A. (1980). Revised, smoothed normative data on the Neuropsychological Test Bettery for Children. Unpublished manuscript.

Leckliter, I.N., Matarazzo, J.D., & Silverstein, A.B. (1986). A literature review of factor analytic studies of the WAIS-R. *Journal of Clinical Psychology, 42,* 3323–3342.

Leckliter, I.N., Forster, A.A., Klonoff, H., & Knights, R.M. (1992). A Review of reference group data from normal children for the Halstead-Reitan Neuropsychological Test Battery for Older Children. *The Clinical Neuropsychologist, 6,* 201–229.

Lehr, E. (1990). *Psychological Management of Traumatic Brain Injuries in Children and Adolescents.* Rockville, MD: Aspen Publishers.

Lezak, M.D. (1983). *Neuropsychological Assessment* (2nd ed.). New York: Oxford University Press.

Luria, A.R. (1980). *Higher cortical functions in man* (2nd ed.). New York: Basic Books.

Matarazzo, J.D. (1990). Psychological assessment versus psychological testing: Validation from Binet to the school, clinic, and classroom. *American Psychologist, 45,* 999–1017.

Rattan, A.I., Rattan, G., Dean, R.S., & Gray, J.W. (1989). Assessing the commonality of the WISC-R and the Halstead-Reitan Neuropsychological test battery with learning-disordered children. *Journal of Psychoeducational Assessment, 7,* 296–303.

Reeder, K.P., & Boll, T.J. (1992). A shortened intermediate version of The Halstead Category Test. *Archives of Clinical Neuropsychology*, *7*, 53–62.

Roid, G.H., Prifitera, A., & Weiss, L.G. (1993). Replication of the WISC-III factor structure in an independent sample. *Journal of Psychoeducational Assessment*, WISC-III Monograph, pp. 6–21.

Rourke, B.P., & Brown, G.G. (1986). Clinical neuropsychology and behavioral neurology: Similarities and differences. In S.B. Filskov & T.J. Boll (Eds.), *Handbook of Clinical Psychology* (Vol. 2, pp. 3–18). New York: Wiley.

Sattler, J.M. (1988). *Assessment of Children (3rd ed.).* San Diego: Author.

Sattler, J.M. (1992). *Assessment of Children: WISC-III and WPPSI-R Supplement.* San Diego: Author.

Sheslow, D., & Adams, W. (1990). *Wide Range Assessment of Memory and Learning: Administration manual.* Wilmington, DE: Jastak Associates.

Strom, D.A., Gray, J.W., Dean, R.S., & Fischer, W.E. (1987). The incremental validity of the Halstead-Reitan Neuropsychological Battery in predicting achieving for learning-disabled children. *Journal of Psychoeducational Assessment, 2,* 157–165.

Swanson, H.L. (1987). Information processing theory and learning disabilities: A commentary and future perspective. *Journal of Learning Disabilities, 20,* 155–166.

Thatcher, R.W. (1991). Maturation of the human frontal lobes: Physiological evidence for staging. *Developmental Neuropsychology, 7,* 397–419.

Wechsler, D.W. (1991). *Manual for the Wechsler Intelligence Scale for Children, Third Edition.* San Antonio: Psychological Corporation.

Welsh, M.C., Pennington, B.F., & Groisser, D.B. (1991). A normative-developmental study of executive function: A window on pre-frontal function in children. *Developmental Neuropsychology, 7,* 131–149.

Wielkiewicz, R.M. (1990). Interpreting low scores on the WISC-R Third Factor: It's more than distractibility. *Journal of Consulting and Clinical Psychology, 2,* 91–97.

CHAPTER 6

Hemispheric Stimulation Techniques in Children with Dyslexia

DIRK J. BAKKER, ROBERT LICHT, and E. JAN KAPPERS

Neuropsychological stimulation of the right or the left hemisphere has been shown to alter the lateral distribution of electrophysiological activity in the brain. It has further been shown that the resultant alterations in electrophysiological activity are correlated with selective improvements in reading. Recently, this stimulation technique has been adopted by a number of learning-disability centers for treating of dyslexic children and underachievers in reading. Before describing these procedures and their relative effectiveness in treating reading-disabled children, we briefly present the rationale for their application.

The Balance Model of Learning to Read and Dyslexia

Theory

Many neuroscientists assume that, in most individuals, disturbances in reading are the result of a malfunction in the left cerebral hemisphere. Because reading is considered a lingual process and such processes have been shown to be mediated by the left hemisphere, the logic in this assumption is apparent. Indeed, lesions of the left hemisphere often result in a language disturbance whereas lesions of the right hemisphere typically do not. But what is meant by the word "lingual?" When it refers to the *phonemic*, *semantic*, and *syntactic* aspects of reading, one should think of predominantly left-hemisphere processes. When "lingual" refers to the form and structure of letters, words, and sentences, however, one may wonder if the left hemisphere is involved in processing these components of reading. The elements of text, the letters, have a form and a left-to-right ordering that can determine the meaning of words and sentences (e.g., name, mane, mean, amen; he is, is he). A change in the lateral ordering of letters in a word or of words in a sentence can result in a change in the meaning of those words and sentences. Letters also have the peculiar quality of changing their meaning depending on their position in space (e.g., p-q, b-d, n-u, m-w) while maintaining their meaning despite changes in their physical shape (e.g., b-B, d-D, p-P). Lateral ordering, spatial position and form, unlike the phonemic, semantic, and syntactic components of reading, are visuo-spatial. Whether reading is predominantly mediated by the right or the left hemisphere depends upon the relative effort required to process each component associated with the text to be read. The novice reader is faced with an array of shapes quite different from those he or she is already familiar with. Because these shapes are unfamiliar, the novice reader must exert substantial effort to analyze these visuo-spatial components. At this stage in learning to read, the reader is primarily engaged in perceptually analyzing text, and so reading is initially subserved predominantly by the right hemisphere. Gradually, as the perceptual analysis of text becomes automatic and drops below the level of consciousness (Fries, 1963), effort is no longer required for such tasks. In the advanced stages of learning to read, syntactic and semantic analyses of text dominate, and these analyses are mediated predominantly by the left hemisphere. Therefore, the balance in effort shifts from the initial analysis of visuo-spatial features to the later analysis of syntactic and semantic features. At the cortical level this shift in the balance of effort is paralleled by a shift in hemispheric mediation of reading. During the initial stages of reading, when perceptual analysis of text predominates, the right hemisphere appears to mediate reading. As reading becomes more advanced with analysis of semantic and syntactic features predominating, the control seems to shift from the right to the left hemisphere. Consequently, as learning to read progresses, a shift in primary hemispheric control will occur.

Predictions by the Balance Model are comparable to those derived from the Novelty Model developed by Goldberg and Costa (1981). These authors argue for right-hemisphere superiority in processing novel information and for left-hemisphere superiority in processing routinized codes and rules. According to this model, reading is mediated by the left hemisphere only when it proceeds according to routinized linguistic rules. Rourke (1982) adds that the "relative salience of the right and left hemisphere systems changes in predictable ways as a function of competence in the various stages of the learning-to-read process" (p. 6). The initial reading stage and parts of the second stage of "'assembling' the units of print (e.g., graphemes) for linkage with the units of the preexisting linguistic systems (e.g., phonemes)" (p. 5), presumably requires predominantly right-hemisphere control.

Evidence

Early investigations into hemispheric control of reading suggested that young children, unlike older children, who showed a strict left-hemisphere pattern of control, displayed a bilateral or right-hemispheric pattern of

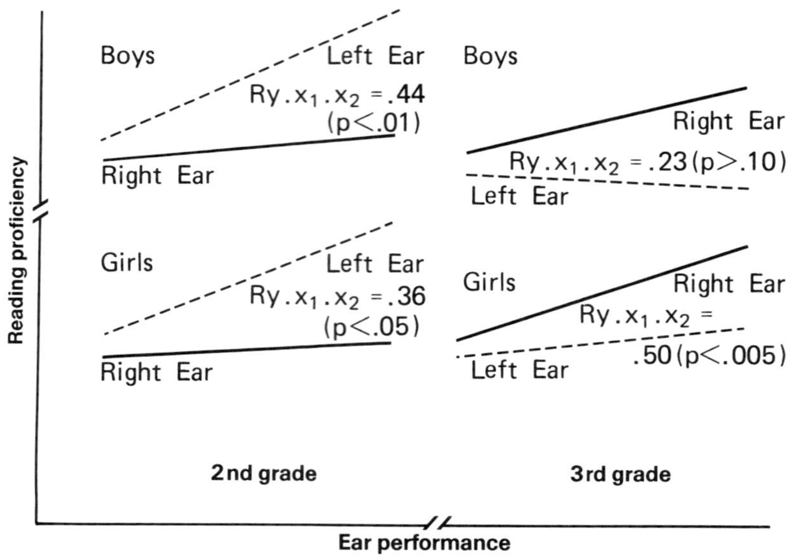

Fig. 6.1. Linear regression of reading proficiency on ear performance by grade, sex, and ear. (Reproduced with permission from Bakker, 1979b.)

control (Bakker, 1973; Bakker, Smink, & Reitsma, 1973). Using verbal listening tasks, reading proficiency was found to correlate with low between-ear differences under verbal dichotic and monaural conditions. Similar findings were reported by Sadick and Ginsburg (1978). It has also been shown that kindergarten children who demonstrate a left-ear advantage (LEA) for verbal information read better in grade 5 than do kindergarten children who demonstrate a right-ear advantage (REA) for verbal information (Bakker, 1979a). Regression of reading proficiency on right- and left-ear recall of verbal auditory inputs in grade 2 and 3 boys and girls is shown in Figure 6.1 (Bakker, 1979b).

Although they indicate that reading proficiency in grades 2 and 3 is associated with increasing left- and right-ear performance respectively, these findings suggest that early reading is predominantly mediated by the right hemisphere but more advanced reading by the left hemisphere. An extensive investigation by Kappers (1986) revealed similar results.

Several visual half-field studies also suggest a developmental shift in hemispheric control of reading. For example, Carmon, Nachshon, & Starinsky (1976) found that older primary-school children demonstrated a right-field advantage (RFA) for verbal inputs but younger primary-school children demonstrated a left-field advantage (LFA) or no advantage for verbal inputs.

A more decisive conclusion can be drawn from a four-year longitudinal electrophysiological investigation of normal children from kindergarten through grade 3 (Licht, 1988; Licht, Bakker, Kok, & Bouma, 1988). These children were asked to read words presented to the central visual field while evoked brain responses (ERPs) were recorded at the left and right temporal and parietal scalp locations. Subjects were also given varied reading- and writing-to-dictation tasks. A principal-component analysis (PC) was performed on the ERP data and a factor analysis (FA) was performed on the scholastic-performance scores. The relationship between the PC and the FA scores revealed a relatively strong association between reading performance and right-hemispheric activity at the first two probes (kindergarten and grade 1) and a relatively strong association between reading performance and the left hemisphere in later probes (see also Bakker, 1990). These findings reinforce the predictions derived from the Balance Model, which posit that control of reading shifts from the right hemisphere to the left during learning to read at the time when perceptual analysis of text becomes automatic and semantic and syntactic analyses of text predominate.

Dyslexia

Knowing that the primary mediation of learning to read normally shifts from one hemisphere to the other, one might suspect that deviations could result in disturbances in acquisition of reading. One can think of a child who for some reason is unable to make the normal right- to left-hemisphere shift during learning to read. We would expect that such a child would continue to rely on right-hemisphere reading strategies. According to the Novelty Model, this child might fail to find and utilize codes and rules necessary to achieve reading fluency. The child would remain focused on the visuo-spatial features of text and thus, would show a slow, fragmented, but relatively accurate style of reading. Dysfunctional readers demonstrating this style have been classified as P-type dyslexics (Bakker, 1979a, 1980, 1992). Another group of children can be found in which the right- to left-hemispheric shift is made too early (these children tend to use left-hemisphere strategies from the very start of learning to read). Because they are not focusing on the surface structure of the text, these children tend to read relatively quickly and produce many substantive errors. Dysfunctional readers demonstrating this reading style have been classified as L-type dyslexics (Bakker, 1979a, 1980, 1992).

The L and P dyslexias are distinguishable by reading speed and accuracy: slow, fragmented reading with relatively high accuracy indicates P-type dyslexia, and fast reading with low accuracy indicates the L type. Although this classification is useful, some dyslexic children cannot be classified in this way. Children who read somewhat slowly with low accuracy or who cannot read at all do not fit within the L and P classification system. By experience we find that approximately 65% of dyslexic children can be classified as either L or P. Some have tried (Bos & van Vliet, 1990) to devise norms based on performance on standardized reading tests to classify dyslexic readers as L, P, or neither. These norms, however, are not valid for languages other than Dutch. A substantial amount of research has been devoted to the correlates of dyslexia and their use in validating the L/P classification system.

Validity of P- and L-Type Dyslexia

Generally, two broad groups of subtyping can be distinguished, named for the theoretical models and classification methods (Hooper & Willis, 1989). The first group, the clinical-inferential approach, defines subtypes according to a theoretical model of reading. Subjects are often classified by only a few test scores. Examples of this approach are among the subtypes described by Boder (1973), Mitterer (1982), Pirozollo (1979), and in the Balance Model (Bakker, 1979a). The second group, using the empirical approach, defines subtypes by advanced statistical methods to increase objectivity (Fletcher & Morris, 1986; Satz & Morrris, 1981). Children are grouped according to similarities in the pattern of their performance profiles by means of Q-factor or cluster analysis. Although several differences appear in the objectivity of the classification procedures used by these approaches, both have the same research goal: to validate the subtypes that are described or extracted.

The typical pattern of errors made by P and L dyslexics is derived by observing reading behavior of children with reading problems. Teachers can pick out the two types of children with relative ease. This facility indicates the clear face validity of the P–L classification system (which is more typical of subtypes described in the clinical-inferential approach than those found by the empirical methods: Hooper & Willis, 1989).

Simply describing or extracting subtypes, though, does not guarantee that these subtypes can be detected reliably or that the classification has validity. First one has to determine the specific characteristics for each subtype and the instruments that will be used to measure these characteristics. Next, one has to show that the subtypes can be classified reliably. If a child is initially classified as a P, this child should be so classified on a second occasion (unless the child has received remediation and thus has changed reading style; we cover this subject in the section on treatment). The validity of subtypes can be determined in several ways: (1) studying subtype X treatment effects; (2) examining subtype differences on variables not used to determine subtypes (e.g., behavioral and electrophysiological variables); (3) examining success in classifying new cases; and (4) comparing the subtypes with those derived from other classifications (Hooper & Willis, 1989). When studying correlates of subtype classifications, expected differences have to be derived from the model on which the subtype classification is based. Thus, if P-type reading is mainly determined by functional overinvolvement by the right hemisphere, one may expect to find fewer errors and faster responses in the left than in the right visual field when words are presented, or electrical indices of relatively higher activity in the right than in the left hemisphere during reading.

Comparisons with Other Subtype Classifications

One way of determining validity is to compare the present L and P classification with those described by other researchers. Boder (1973) classifies dyslexic children in dyseidetic, dysphonetic, and mixed subtypes. Dyseidetic subjects have difficulty in using visual whole-word information in reading and perform poorly on irregular words. They are relatively normal in applying grapheme and phoneme rules, however. Dysphonetic dyslexics, though, have trouble using grapheme-phoneme rules and have to rely on their sight-word vocabulary when recognizing words. The dyslexic subtypes distinguished by Mitterer (1982)—recoding and whole-word readers—are very similar to Boder's dyseidetic and dysphonetic subtypes. These classification systems are based on deficiencies in using the indirect (phonological) or direct (lexical) routes for word recognition as put forward in the dual-access model of reading (Barron, 1986).

Because P and L dyslexics are classified according to substantive and time-consuming (fragmentation) reading errors, several studies have been undertaken to compare P and L dyslexics on measures of different strategies in word recognition (Bakker, Licht, & Van Strien, 1991; Licht, 1989; Van Strien, Bouma, & Bakker, 1993).

In one of the first studies, a word-decoding task (WDT) consisting of regular, irregular, and pseudowords was presented to P and L children. They were also presented with the Stroop color-interference task (STROOP) and a reading task (READ), with a standard reading condition and an auditory and visual noise condition. Results indicated that L dyslexics were generally faster than P dyslexics and made relatively more errors in the WDT on pseudowords than on irregular words, whereas P children showed the reverse pattern of errors (see Table 6.1).

Both auditory and visual noise also slowed reading speed in P-types, but only visual noise slowed it in L-types. Finally, L-types showed a larger increase in color-naming time than did P-types, presumably because of interference by the words presented in the STROOP. Together these findings suggest that L readers tend to rely on a direct visual word-recognition strategy, but P children prefer an indirect, phonological strategy (Licht, 1989). This reading strategy preferred by L and P children was replicated by Neijens (1991) using the WDT. The direct

Table 6.1. Number of errors in the WDT and reading time in the STROOP and READ task for P- and L-type dyslexics.

Licht	WDT			STROOP			READ		
(1989)	R	I	P	A	B	C	S	A	V
P-type (29)	9.5	20.0	15.1	100	104	193	152	170	195
L-type (28)	5.5	10.0	14.8	75	104	220	115	115	137
Neijens (1991)									
P-type (14)	7.5	17.9	14.1						
L-type (9)	7.3	12.6	15.4						

Note: Number of subjects in parentheses. WDT: R = regular, I = irregular, P = pseudo; STROOP: A = color naming, B = word reading, C = naming color of words; READ: S = standard, A = auditory noise, V = visual noise.

strategy is associated with fast reading, whereas the phonological or indirect strategy is associated with slow and more elaborate reading.

If we compare P and L dyslexics with the subtypes distinguished by Boder and Mitterer, we find that the P is most similar to the dyseidetic and the recoding subtype, whereas the L can be equated with the dysphonetic and the whole-word subtype.

In a follow-up study we tried to determine whether differences between P and L children in word-recognition strategy could be attributed to differences in the speed and accuracy with which they visually analyzed words, or to differences at a higher, lexical level of processing, or both. We presented L and P children and normal readers with tasks based on the component approach described by Frederiksen (1980). In this approach, different tasks either tap specific stages in word recognition (e.g., visual, phonological, lexical, or semantical analysis), or require specific responses (e.g., reading aloud or decision making).

These tasks were presented: (1) a simple reaction-time task (BRT), which provided a measure of basic response speed; (2) a visual-scanning task (VSCAN), which required the child to determine if all the letters in a four-letter array were visually similar; (3) a letter-identification task (LIDEN) in which the child had to decide whether all letters in a four-letter array had the same name identity (letter arrays consisted of combinations of lower- and upper-case letters); (4) a lexical decision (LEX) task that required the child to determine whether a presented word was a real Dutch word or a pseudoword; and (5) a semantic decision task (SEM) in which the child had to decide whether or not a word was an animal name. It was expected that P children, relying on a phonological/indirect strategy, would show longer response times in the lexical and semantic tasks, relative to the simpler letter-scanning and identity tasks. The L dyslexics, employing a whole-word reading strategy, were expected to show more errors in the letter-scanning and identity tasks relative to the lexical and semantic tasks that would be faster.

Table 6.2. Mean response times and standard deviations for P- and L-type dyslexics and normal readers.

	BRT	LSCAN	LIDEN	LEXD	SEMD
P-type	339 (97)	981 (178)	1,471 (336)	2,099 (552)	1,569 (412)
L-type	342 (97)	1,133 (187)	1,694 (272)	1,803 (421)	1,495 (346)
Normals	369 (111)	947 (148)	1323 (248)	1,277 (288)	1,015 (198)

Analyzing response times and error scores (see Table 6.2) revealed: (1) no differences between P and L children and normal readers in basic response time (BRT); (2) L children were slower than P children and normal readers on letter-scanning and letter-identity tasks, whereas P-types were slower than normal readers only on the letter-identity task; (3) normal readers were faster than both P and L children on the lexical- and semantic-decision tasks, whereas L types were faster than P types when making lexical decisions; P children were particularly slow on pseudowords in the lexical-decision task; and (4) P and L dyslexics made more errors than normal readers on the letter-identity and lexical-decision tasks and on the animal names within the semantic-decision task; P children made more errors on pseudowords than on normal words in the lexical task. These findings suggest that L children have problems when a letter-by-letter analysis is required, but when a whole-word analysis is required, they switch to a fast, direct-reading strategy. The P children seem to have problems when lexical access and lexical search is required, as reflected in their performance on the pseudowords in the lexical-decision task. These problems cannot, however, be attributed to deficits in visual analysis of letter strings, for their performance is comparable to that of normals and superior to that of L types on these tasks (Licht, in press). In studies by Van Strien (Van Strien, Bakker, Bouma, & Koops, 1988) similar differences between L and P dyslexics have been reported. These authors found that L children performed less well than P children and normal readers on a task that required children to rotate figures mentally. Because this task calls upon ability to discriminate between shapes, it was concluded that L-type children have specific difficulties in processing visuo-spatial (text) features. The L and P dyslexics and normal readers were also given a lexical-decision task consisting of three- and four-letter words and pseudowords. All groups showed longer response times on four- than on three-letter pseudowords, whereas P children also showed this effect with words. In addition, P children took longer to respond to pseudowords than to normal words relative to L children and normal readers (see Table 6.3). These findings support our previous conclusion that P children rely on a slow, phonological/indirect-reading strategy and that they appear to have problems in accessing or searching their lexicon. The L children, like normal readers, tend to use a direct-reading strategy when reading familiar words.

Table 6.3. Mean response times of P- and L-type dyslexics and normal readers in a lexical decision task with 3- and 4-letter words and nonwords.

	Words		Nonwords	
	3	4	3	4
P-type	1,863	1,978	2,427	2,802
L-type	1,661	1,637	1,956	2,272
Normals	1,029	1,014	1,130	1,214

Source: From Van Strien et al. (1993), with permission.

In word-decoding and visuo-spatial skills, P and L dyslexics look similar to the auditory-linguistic subtype and the visual-spatial subtype respectively, described by Pirozollo (1979). Data on performance in different functional areas are not available, however, and so neuropsychological profiles of P and L children with the subtypes distinguished by Pirozollo cannot yet be compared.

Differences in Attention Between P- and L-Type Dyslexics

Behavioral Measures

In further validation studies of the P and L classification, we examined whether P and L dyslexics could be differentiated from each other and from normal readers on tasks that required selective or sustained allocation of attention. It is generally found that reading disability is associated with disturbances in attention (August & Garfinkel, 1990; Dykman & Ackerman, 1991). The finding that L children benefited more than P children from hemisphere-specific stimulation (HSS; Bakker & Vinke, 1985), a neuropsychological treatment method that is described extensively in the paragraph on experimental treatment procedures, was one of the main reasons for instigating the study of attentional differences between P and L children. The HSS method requires the child to fixate on a central point on a television screen while attention is allocated to either the left or right visual field. Words are then flashed briefly to either the right or the left visual field and the child is asked to read these words. It was hypothesized that differences in ability to direct attention to spatial fields and/or to sustain attention during task performance might underlie HSS's differential treatment effects of P and L dyslexics. In one of the first studies, P and L children were asked to differentiate target shapes from background shapes, letters, or (pseudo)words in the Revised Underlining Test (Rourke & Petraukas, 1977). It was found that L types were as accurate as P types on shape and letter targets but they were more accurate than P dyslexics when the targets were (pseudo)words (Licht,

1989). In a study by Neijens (De Sonneville, Neijens, & Licht, 1993) a computerized Bourdon task was given to P and L children. This task requires that the child press a left-response button when a three- or five-dot pattern is presented (nontargets) and a right-response button when a four-dot pattern is presented (targets). All dot patterns are presented to the center of a television screen. Although both P and L children appeared to be slower than normal controls on the four-dot patterns, the dyslexic children showed fluctuation in response times across trials compared with the normal group, perhaps indicating a deficit in sustained attention (see Figure 6.2a). Differences between L and P children were limited to the number of misses on the four-dot patterns: L types showed an increase in the number of misses, and P children showed a more consistent pattern of misses during task performance (Figure 6.2b). The latter finding suggests a decline in vigilance in L children during the task.

It was also found that both P and L dyslexics had higher hyperactivity and inattention scores on the Child Behavior Check List compared to norms for their age, as rated by parents and teachers (CBCL; Verhulst, Koot, Akkerhuis, & Veerman, 1990). The ratings were higher for L than for P children, but these differences did not reach significance.

Leek (1993; De Sonneville, Leek, & Licht, in preparation) replicated the dot-pattern attention task (De Sonneville, 1993) and extended it by adding divided- and focused-attention tasks. Again dyslexic children, compared to normal controls, showed larger fluctuations in response times across trials on the dot-pattern task. An increase in misses on four-dot patterns during task performance was also found, but no differences were found between P and L children. The focused-attention task required the children to respond with a "yes" button only to target letters presented at the relevant diagional of the display and to respond with a "no" button to all other stimuli (nontargets and all letters presented at the irrelevant diagonal). Both P and L children displayed longer response time to nontargets than to targets presented at the relevant diagonal, suggesting that both subtypes were able to use a focused-attention strategy. In the divided-attention task the child was asked to respond with a "yes" button when presented with target letters and with a "no" button when target letters were absent. One or three target letters (memory load) could be presented in a display with letters. The letters could be intact or visually degraded. This task is based on the additive-factor model (AFM) of Sternberg (1969) and enables us to investigate speed and accuracy at different stages in information processing. Stimulus quality (intact vs. degraded) would influence only the stage of stimulus encoding, whereas the number of targets (one vs. three) and the type of response (yes vs. no) would influence the stage in memory search and the stage in decision making, respectively.

In general, longer response times were found for degraded letters, for "no" responses, and for three target letters in the display. Overall, P

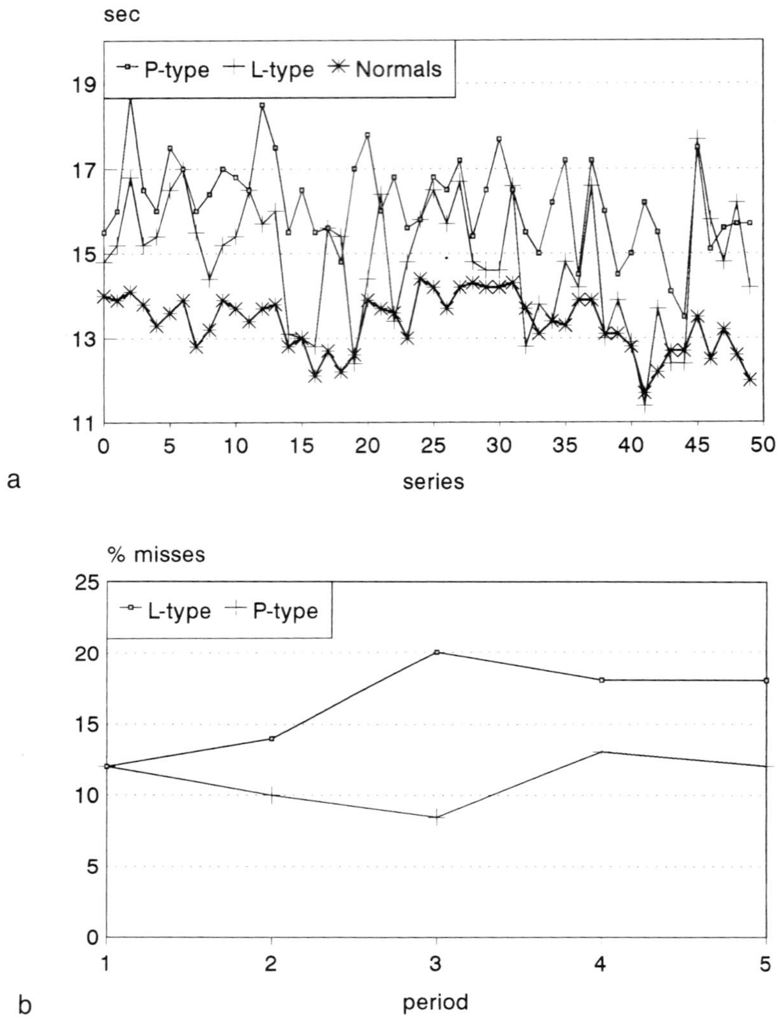

Fig. 6.2. (a) Mean response times for P- and L-type dyslexics and normals in the dot pattern task, depicted as a function of series. Each series consisted of 12 trials. (b) Average percentage of errors (4 dot patterns) for P- and L-type dyslexics as a function of period (a period consisted of 10 series). (After Neijens, 1991.)

children were slower than L children. The finding that P dyslexics had larger differences, between "yes" and "no" responses than L dyslexics suggests that P children have a delay in the stage of decision making. This effect was also more pronounced when degraded nontarget letters were presented in the one-target condition. The latter finding is somewhat puzzling and may indicate that in dyslexic children and particularly in P children the letter has to be encoded several times before memory search and decision making can be completed.

Electrocortical Measures of Attention, Reading, and Hemispheric Involvement

The behavioral studies on validity of the P- and L-type classification, were added to by several studies using brain electrical activity as a dependent variable. These experiments investigate the differential hemispheric involvement in P and L children during processing of words and during attention-demanding tasks. One advantage in measuring electrical brain activity is that it can be recorded during task performance from many electrode locations on the head. Unlike the more traditional test approach or reaction-time tasks focused on the "end product," the recording of event-related potentials (ERPs) enables us to study the energetic or computational aspects of stimulus processing.

Attention

One of the first studies analyzed ERPs elicited during a word-reading task, in P and L dyslexics, and was administered at the beginning and end of a treatment program (Bakker, Moerland, & Goekoop-Hoefkens, 1981; Bakker & Vinke, 1985). Difference-ERPs (posttreatment-pretreatment) reported in the Bakker & Vinke study showed an increase in negativity in the period around 200 to 250 ms. These amplitude changes were most pronounced in L dyslexics who received HSS and appeared to be correlated with an increase in reading accuracy. The finding that HSS affected the amplitude of relatively early peaks in the ERP suggests that treatment had either increased processing efficiency in the early stages of word analysis or brought about a change in allocation of energy (attention) to these early processing stages, or a combination of both. Hillyard (1984) provides additional evidence for the finding that the amplitudes of early ERP peaks are sensitive to attentional manipulations. Behavioral measures of attention, discussed in the preceding section, revealed that P and particularly L dyslexics showed defects in sustaining their attention, reflected in response fluctuations. Because one of our research questions was whether P and L children differed from each other in their ability to direct attention to relevant spatial locations and to selectively process stimuli designated as targets, ERPs were recorded during a selective-attention and a spatial-cueing task. The selective-attention task required the child to respond to a target letter only when it was presented at a relevant location (either the left or right visual field in a block of trials), and to refrain from responding to all other letters and all letters presented at irrelevant locations. In selective-attention research it has been found that selecting stimulus location is associated with increased amplitudes of

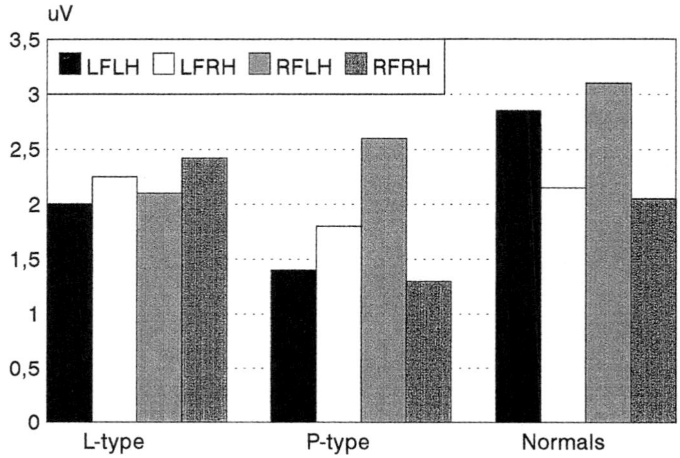

Fig. 6.3. Amplitudes (attended-unattended) of the late positive potential (P500) over the left and right hemisphere for right- and left-field presentations in P- and L-type dyslexics and normal readers. (LFLH = left visual field–left hemisphere; LFRH = left visual field–right hemisphere; RFLH = right visual field–left hemisphere; RFRH = right visual field–right hemisphere)

early negative or positive waves over contralateral sites (N1 effect), whereas selecting of target stimuli presented at the relevant location elicits large positive potentials (P300 effect) over parietal areas. In our study we also found increased negativity over parietal sites contralateral to the relevant field, but no group differences appeared in hemispheric distribution of this attention-related negativity. The L children showed larger negativity than P children at frontal locations, whereas P children and normal readers had larger positivity at occipital locations than L dyslexics. Tentatively, these findings suggest differential involvement of frontal and posterior brain areas in spatial orienting in P and L children. Both P and L children and normal readers showed increased positive potentials at parietal locations for relevant targets, indicating that the dyslexics have no problem in selecting target letters from a series of background letters. The groups of children differed, however, in hemispheric distribution of this late positivity as a function field. Normal readers showed consistently larger amplitudes over the left than over the right hemisphere, whereas L children had smaller amplitudes that were somewhat larger over the right than over the left hemisphere. The P children showed larger amplitudes over the left than over the right hemisphere for right-field presentations and the reverse with much smaller amplitudes for left-field presentations (see Figure 6.3). The functional significance of these amplitude differences is not yet clear, for no significant differences appeared between the dyslexic groups at the behavioral level. In any case, the pattern of hemispheric asymmetries shows differential involvement by left and right hemispheres in P and L dyslexics

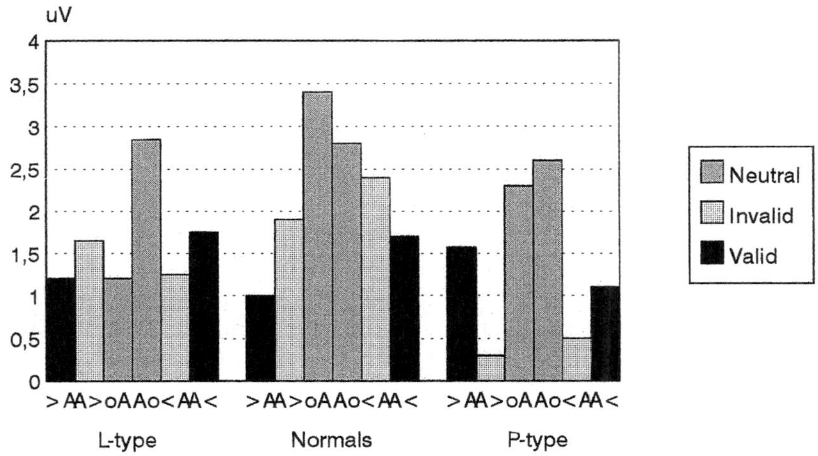

Fig. 6.4. Average amplitudes in the period of 100–200 ms elicited by the reaction stimulus on neutral, valid and invalid trials in P- and L-type dyslexics and normal readers. > indicates direction of arrow cue, o indicates the neutral cue. (With permission from Jonkman et al., © 1992 Lawrence Gilbaum Associates, Inc.)

during processing of letter stimuli (Licht, Jonkman, Bakker, & Woestenburg, 1990). The second study on attentional differences between P and L children employed a cueing task developed by Posner (1978). In this task a centrally presented arrow, pointing to the left or right visual field, cues the location for the possible appearance of a reaction stimulus. An attentional set was created by making 75% of the trials valid—i.e., the reaction stimulus was presented at the cued location. In control conditions a circle was presented as a cue, indicating a 50% chance that the reaction stimulus would be presented in the right or in the left field and a number of "catch" trials, consisting of an arrow only, were interspersed. In contrast with the selective-attention task, in which a field was relevant during a whole block of trials, the subject now had to select the relevant location on each trial. On a behavioral level it was found that, for all groups, valid trials resulted in faster responses than did invalid trials, confirming the idea that cueing directed attention to the location where the reaction stimulus would appear. It was further found that arrows pointing to the left elicited larger amplitudes over the right posterior locations in the period from 100 to 600 ms after presentation, whereas right arrows showed similar effects in the period from 450 to 600 ms, but larger amplitudes over the left posterior sites for earlier periods. Circles tended to show the same pattern as left arrows. These findings confirm the notion that right-posterior brain areas are involved in orienting and directing attention to different spatial locations (Heilman & Van den Abel, 1979). The P and L children did not differ from normal readers in these amplitude effects, suggesting that orienting and shifting of attention is normal in these children. Presenting the reaction stimulus, however, elicited a positive peak that was differentially affected by the validity of the information (on the cued location or on the uncued location) in the P and L group and in normal readers. The P children showed larger amplitudes on valid than on invalid trials, whereas normal readers showed the opposite pattern. The L children showed consistently larger amplitudes when the reaction stimulus was presented in the left visual field, regardless of the direction of the preceding cue (see Figure 6.4).

As with the selective-attention task, no differences in error pattern or response times were found between P and L children, complicating interpretation of the found ERP effects in terms of functional differences. It seems, however, that brain areas in both P children and normal readers differentiate between letters presented at cued or uncued locations, whereas in L children, brain activity differentiates only between locations of the letter stimulus (Jonkman, Licht, Bakker, & Van den Broek-Sandmann, 1992).

Reading

In a study conducted in conjunction with the research group of the University of Jyväskylä (Finland), a probe paradigm was used to assess hemispheric activation in P and L children while different texts were read. The probe paradigm consisted of presenting a primary task, to which the subject had to attend. During performance, task-irrelevant probe stimuli (tones or light flashes or both) were presented, and evoked potentials were recorded for these presentations (probe stimuli). It is assumed that brain regions involved in the primary task will show smaller responses to the probe stimuli because of their limited capacity for processing. In the present study four conditions were introduced: reading silently, reading aloud, reading visually loaded text, and an arithmetic task. Preliminary findings for the silent-reading condition show that L children have larger amplitudes than P children for an early negative wave (N100) at frontal-central locations elicited by probe tones. In contrast, P children have larger amplitudes than L children for a similar wave at the same locations when a visual probe is presented. These findings may indicate group differences in the balance between phonological and visual processes in reading. Further analysis of the data is necessary, however, to reveal the validity of the findings (Aro, Licht, & Lyytinen, 1993).

In conclusion, classifying reading-disabled children as P- or L-type dyslexic by their pattern of reading errors and reading speed seems valid behaviorally as well as electrophysiologically. On a behavioral level, several studies show that L children differ from P children in word-recognition strategy, mental rotation, and ability to sustain attention. In word-reading strategies, P and L children can be equated with subtypes described by Boder (1973), Mitterer (1982), and Pirozollo (1979). Electrophysiologically it was found that P and L children showed different patterns of hemispheric activation during reading and processing of letters, indicating differential involvement of left- and right-brain areas.

Experimental Treatment Procedures and Outcomes

Rationale

For P-type dyslexic children, those who presumably fail to shift from the right to the left hemisphere in generating reading strategies, reading should benefit from stimulation of the left hemisphere and reading by L-type dyslexics should benefit from right-hemisphere stimulation. If the predicted effects on reading are found, we anticipate that these findings will correlate with stimulation-induced alterations in lateral distribution of hemispheric activity. This prediction implies that the brain can be permanently changed in response to environmental stimulation. For this implication, we refer the reader to a large body of research showing that a number of neural parameters undergo lasting change as a result of increased environmental stimulation (learning) (see Renner & Rosenzweig, 1987; for a survey see Bakker, 1989). These studies provide the rationale for assuming that stimulating the left hemisphere in P dyslexics and the right hemisphere in L dyslexics should bring about alterations in the hemispheric substrate of reading, which would in turn underlie changes in reading performance.

Procedures

Hemisphere stimulation can be accomplished in two ways: (1) hemisphere-specific stimulation (HSS) or (2) hemisphere-alluding stimulation (HAS).

The HSS technique provides for presenting reading material to the right or the left visual field (HSS-vis), to the right or the left ear (HSS-aud), and/or to the fingers of the right or the left hand (HSS-tac) in P and L dyslexics, respectively. The right visual field and the right hand project onto the left hemisphere, whereas the reverse holds true for the left visual field and the left hand. This dissociation in hemispheric projection is not total in the auditory channel, however, where ipsilateral projections exist but contralateral projections dominate. To reduce activation of the ipsilateral hemisphere during auditory presentations, one might present verbal information to one ear (words), simultaneously presenting nonverbal information (instrumental music) to the other ear. In HSS-vis the subject is asked to fixate on a point at the middle of a television screen and is subsequently asked to read words flashed either to the right (P type) or to the left (L type) of this central fixation point. The HEMSTIM (note 1) computer program generates HSS-vis (Moerland & Bakker, 1993). This program, which runs on IBM XT and AT machines employing the MS-DOS operating system, consists of three integrated modules: (1) a stimulus-preparation and editing module, (2) a training module, and (3) a database-manipulation and reporting module. Within the training module, these parameters can be modified: (1) letter font, (2) stimulus file, (3) exposure time, (4) foreground and background colors, (5) reading task, (6) cursor shape and mouse sensitivity, (7) speed of automatic mouse cursor moves, and (8) difficulty of the fixation task. In HSS-vis, the child is required to fuse a floating mouse cursor with a central target on the screen. Fusion of the cursor and the target is followed by one or two words flashed in one of the visual half-fields. The subject is typically asked to read these words aloud and may be required to perform other tasks simultaneously (e.g., matching the two words).

The HSS-aud technique may be considered an addendum to HSS-vis and HSS-tac in that the subject's own voice and the voice of the trainer, via a microphone and headphones, are relayed to the right (P-types) or the left (L-types) ear while instrumental music is played in the other ear (Bakker, 1990).

The HSS-tac method is accomplished by presenting words in a tactile training box (see Figure 6.5). The (plastic) letters that form the words and sentences are fastened to the grooves of the planning board. The material to be read is presented, out of sight, to the fingers of the right (P) or the left (L) hand (Bakker, 1990).

The HAS technique provides for presenting ordinary school text, adapted so that presentation alludes to either left- or right-hemispheric processing. Children with P dyslexia are asked to read passages that are made phonetically and semantically complex by omitting words that have to be found by the subject using rhyme or context (Figure 6.6; Bakker, 1990). Children with L dyslexia are presented with perceptually demanding text.

The computer program SCRAMBLER (Note 1) can generate text in any mixture of typefaces (Figure 6.7); mixing typefaces within words increases the perceptual difficulty of the task. Text that is perceptually complex presumably is processed primarily by the right hemisphere (Bakker, 1990).

The HSS and HAS methods provide for unilateral and bilateral presentation of reading material, respectively, to stimulate the right or the

[1]The MS-DOS versions of the computer programs HEMSTIM and SCRAMBLER, as well as the tactile training box, are commercially available from: Information Technology Center for the Handicapped (CIG); Patrijsweg 36; 2289 EX Rijswijk (ZH); Netherlands (FAX . . . 70-3191305).

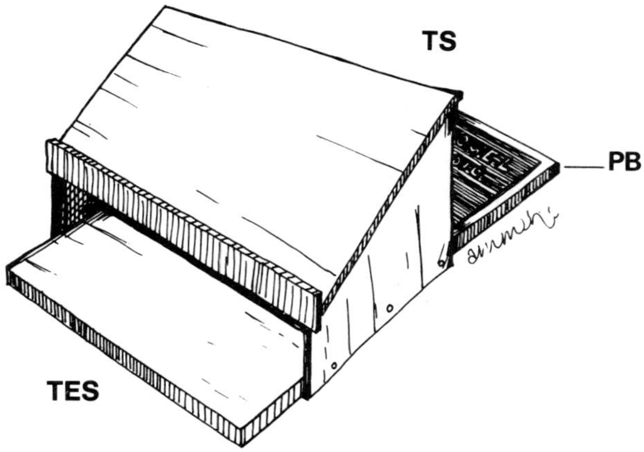

Fig. 6.5. Tactile training box. PB, planning board; TS, trainer's side; TES, trainee's side. (With permission from Bakker, 1990.)

left hemisphere either directly or indirectly. The HAS version was developed at the request of teachers who required a treatment method that was transferable to a classroom situation, because HSS was not.

Of course it is possible to administer combined HSS and HAS techniques, either within or between treatment sessions, for one technique may serve as a catalyst for the other (Bakker, Spyer, & Hoekman, 1990; Russo, 1993; see also the section on outpatient dyslexics). It is also possible to coordinate use of the HSS program for treatment in a specialized institute and use of the HAS program for treatment within the regular classroom.

LINES AND SQUARES

Whenever I walk in a London street,
I'm ever so careful to watch my ________;
    And I keep in the squares,
    And the masses of bears,
Who wait at the corners all ready to eat
The sillies who tread on the lines of the street
    Go back to their lairs,
    And I say to them, "Bears,
    Just look how I'm ________ in all of the squares!"

Fig. 6.6. Hemisphere-alluding stimulation (HAS); can be used in P-type dyslexia. (With permission from Bakker, 1990.)

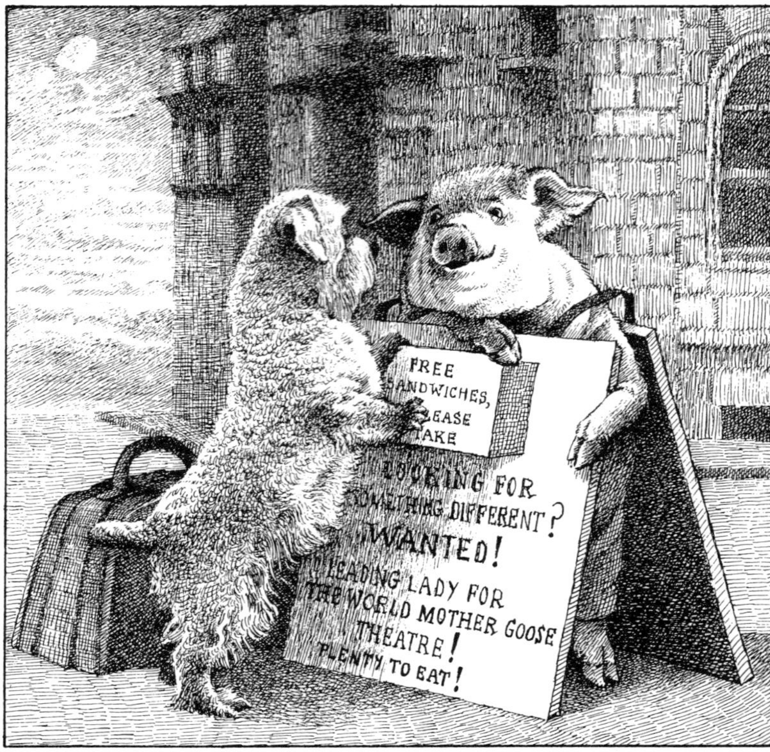
FREE
ANDWICHES,
EASE
AKE
FOR
DIFFERENT?
WANTED!
LADY FOR
MOTHER GOOSE
THEATRE!
TO EAT!

Jennie took everything and went out into the world. On the corner she met a small pig wearing large sandwich boards. He smiled and pointed to a box attached to the front board on which was printed: Free sandwiches, Please Take. Jennie chose a tuna on rye and gobbled it as she read the advertisement on the board.

Fig. 6.7. Hemisphere-alluding stimulation (HAS); can be used in L-type dyslexia. (With permission from Bakker, 1990.)

Both HSS and HAS assume that the child is at least able to name letters. The child who does not have this ability must be trained before either program can be initiated (Kappers & Hamburger, in press).

Stimulating the left hemisphere (P-types) is predicted to enhance fluency of reading (increased speed and decreased fragmentation). This effect, initially, may negatively affect accuracy with a resultant increase in substantive errors. Stimulating the right hemisphere (L-types) is predicted to improve accuracy of reading and to lower reading speed.

Outcomes

Early research began with a pilot study (Bakker, Moreland, & Goekoop-Hoefkins, 1981). This investigation suggested that HSS-vis, compared to placebo and control treatments, altered the lateral distribution of electrophysiological activity within the brain and selectively improved reading performance in both L and P dyslexic children.

In a more extensive study by Bakker and Vinke (1985), L and P dyslexic children received HSS-vis, HAS, or a control treatment. Compared to the control condition, HSS-vis produced changes in the right–left distribution of brain activity. In reading efficiency, as measured with standardized tests, HSS-vis was more effective with L dyslexics and HAS was more effective with P dyslexics (Bakker & Vinke, 1985). The effect of HSS-vis in L dyslexics was reflected in a posttreatment decrease in substantive reading errors and speed. An interesting finding (according to personal communications with fellow researchers working in this area) is the positive effect of HSS-vis on the reading of flashed words in P dyslexics. This effect may indicate treatment-induced enhancement of processing speed in the left hemisphere. All results mentioned were achieved in 22 weekly sessions of about 30 minutes each.

In a field experiment conducted by Bakker, Bouma, & Gardien (1990) with more than 50 remedial-reading teachers as trainers, both P and L dyslexic children received either HSS-tac or a control treatment (20 sessions, 2 per week for about 45 minutes a session). Relative to the control condition, HSS-tac was shown to be effective in enhancing reading fluency in children with P-type dyslexia.

As we have stated, HSS and HAS can be combined effectively within one treatment program. In fact this combination happens implicitly when HSS-vis is employed in treating L-dyslexia; in this situation the words that are flashed in the left visual field (HSS-vis) are made perceptually demanding (HAS) by mixing typefaces. Another HSS-HAS combination investigated by Van Strien, Stolk, & Zuiker (in press) flashes words with negative emotional loading (i.e., pain, dagger) to the lateral visual fields of L and P dyslexics. Evidence says that threatening stimuli activate the right hemisphere (Van Strien & Morpurgo, 1992). Reading in L dyslexics seems to improve significantly more after treatment with emotional words than with neutral words. It would be valuable to learn about the utility of these various treatment techniques in non-Dutch languages. Three experimental studies have been conducted, two with English-speaking children and another with Finnish-speaking children.

Grace (Grace & Spreen, in press) conducted a pilot study followed by a major investigation that methodologically replicated the work of Bakker and Vinke (1985). In the pilot study, groups of L and P dyslexic children were given either HSS-vis or a control treatment for twelve sessions, which took place three times per week for approximately 45 minutes each. The pilot-study results replicated findings by Bakker and Vinke (1985) on the effects of HSS-vis on hemispheric activity and reading performance. The results of the larger follow-up study, however were at odds with those of the pilot study and those of the Bakker and Vinke (1985) study. In this study, HSS-vis relative to the control condition for L dyslexics decreased reading accuracy. In the attempt to explain this unexpected result it was shown that the tasks employed to stimulate the right hemisphere of L dyslexics in fact enhanced electrophysiological activity in the left hemisphere. Thus, the unexpected finding is less surprising but raises the question of how right-hemisphere stimulation could increase left-hemisphere activity. A possible answer may lie in the fixation targets used in the experiment. Grace used symbols like "%" and "&" as targets. These are common figures that are easily coded verbally. The verbal coding, however, may have primed the left hemisphere, and this priming may have overidden activation of the right hemisphere. The idea of priming motivated development of a new experimental option in the HEMSTIM program. In the new option, both the cursor and the fixation target can be made verbal (letters) or nonverbal (faces) to prime the left or the right hemisphere respectively, and these primes then precede the lateral presentation of words.

In a study by Russo (1993), left-handed L-type underachievers in reading were randomly divided into three conditions: (1) (E)xperimental: HSS-vis followed by HSS-tac; (2) (P)lacebo: word games; or (3) (C)ontrol: received routine educational services. Experimental training lasted 14 weeks and consisted of three 15-minute sessions per week. The E children showed marked treatment-induced decrease in substantive reading errors (65%; reported power >0.98, at $p < 0.05$) and the P and C children improved by 9.8% and 1.7% respectively. In reading comprehension, E children improved 33.3%, P children improved 16.0%, and C children improved 22.0%. No significant effect of HSS was found in word identification. Because the word-identification test is reported to capitalize on the speed with which words are identified, positive effect of treatment was not anticipated.

Neuvonen, Rekio-Viinikainen, Ahonen, & Lyytinen (1992) did multiple single-case studies with native Finnish-speaking children with L and P dyslexias. Experimental subjects received HSS-vis twice a week, 30 minutes each time. The entire experiment consisted of 16 sessions given in two blocks of 8 sessions each. Control subjects received remedial teaching for the same period. All experimental L and P dyslexic children are reported to have improved more, on all measures of reading ability, than any of the control children.

In conclusion, the results of the various investigations presented here show that neuropsychological treatment of L and P dyslexic children may be beneficial. Questions remain, however, about the durability of such treatment effects, because very little experimental information is currently available (see also the last section in this chapter).

Because the neuropsychological treatments discussed here have been in practical use at the Paedological Institute Out-Patient Department for Learning Disabled Children for some time, we discuss clinical cases in the remainder of this chapter. The services of the Out-Patient Department are supported by the Netherlands Health Insurance Fund in cases of severe dyslexia.

Neuropsychological Treatment of Dyslexic Outpatients

An outpatient department was founded at the Paedological Institute in Amsterdam to convert scientific knowledge about dyslexia into treatments and to carry out clinical intervention research on these treatments.

We discuss next some of the problems encountered in translating scientific theory and experimental evidence into everyday practice of treatment. We illustrate the latter treatment practices with two case studies.

Although Bakker (1986, 1990) has already made the jump from neuropsychological theory to the treatment of P- and L-types of dyslexia, problems remain that must be solved before such treatments can be done. The translation from theory into practice is more complex than might be assumed. Many implicit decisions are made and many explicit decisions have to be made that are not always inherent in the original theory (Kappers, 1993).

First, a clinician is faced with "every type of dyslexia." After diagnosing a child as dyslexic, the clinician often must conclude that it is not a pure P-type, a pure L-type, or a mixed type. Whether the child can be classified or not, the therapist must accept the child for treatment.

Second, the treatment methods devised by Bakker (1990), require that the child be able to read at a "minimum" level. Initially dyslexic children, however, cannot read at a level that is sufficient to profit from these treatment methods. What then can be done for these children from a neuropsychological perspective?

Third, a clinician is sometimes faced with a dyslexic child who is found, during the diagnostic examination, to have related neurological dysfunctions or even brain damage. According to some definitions of dyslexia (Dumont, 1990), such children would not be classified as dyslexic, but from a neuropsychological perspective they are an intriguing treatment group.

Fourth, in some cases of severe dyslexia, the clinician is faced with a "continuous" problem. The continuity of this problem, among others, is the result of the severe dyslexic child's need for extensive repetition before generalization can be achieved. For example, after an "L(-like) type" is successfully treated, the child may read accurately but too slowly and make numerous time-consuming (fragmentation) errors. Does this child, who now resembles a "P(-like) type," need left-hemispheric stimulation to enhance reading fluency? When and from what evidence does one commence such alternative training techniques?

A final problem is choosing treatment materials. Bakker, from a neuropsychological point of view, suggests how the clinician can: (1) decide which hemisphere should be stimulated, (2) devise methods to carry out the treatment, and (3) enhance the appeal of the stimulation by tailoring the stimuli to the identified functions of the chosen hemisphere. An example of the latter is use of perceptually complex letters in a word that is presented to the left visual half field. Taking into account the great variability among dyslexic children in reading competency and age, the above-mentioned methods cannot at once be put into everyday practice. One must first answer questions about appropriateness of stimuli to level of difficulty, considering (1) language used, (2) orthographic presentation, and (3) level of reading task.

From Assessment to Treatment

Now that the questions about developing appropriate treatments have been raised, how do we go about finding the answers? From our experience, the search should focus on the phased sequence followed in learning to read proposed by the Balance Model and the Novelty Model (Goldberg & Costa, 1981), and thus will not focus primarily on classifying dyslexia. We feel too that elements of information-processing theory should be incorporated into treatment procedures.

Remembering that learning to read is done in phases, we find that according to both models initial reading is primarily mediated by the right hemisphere (RH) and advanced reading is primarily mediated by the left hemisphere (LH). Having this knowledge, the first question we must ask before starting any treatment program is: In which developmental phase of reading does the problem lie?

To answer this question, one must determine at which reading level the child has stagnated. For problems at the initial level, one can hypothesize that there will be a resultant hypofunctioning of the right cerebral hemisphere. In these cases, specific stimulation of the right hemisphere should be carried out. In cases with preinitial (subskill level) reading problems, right-hemisphere stimulation is also thought to be effective in facilitating reading. If reading problems are found at an advanced level, the type of reading strategy used by the child, which Bakker describes as typical for cases of unbalanced hemispheric mediation, should be examined. Is a hasty, inaccurate reading style—plagued with excessive substantive (su) errors (additions, omissions, mutations)—dominant? If this is the style, one can suppose that premature mediation of the reading process by the LH has occurred and RH stimulation is advised. If the dominant reading strategy is slow and accurate, however, with excessive time-consuming (tc) errors (fragmentations), the condition would point to hyperfunctioning of the RH in mediation of reading, and LH stimulation would be advised.

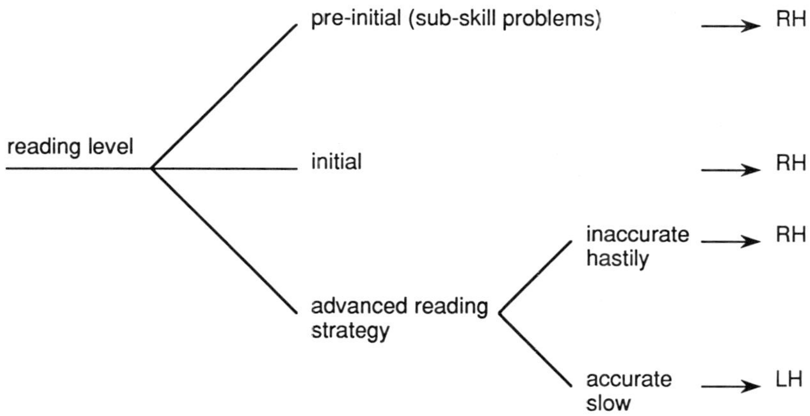

Fig. 6.8. A decision tree for deciding which hemisphere should be stimulated according to the "balance and novelty models" (from: Kappers & Hamburger, in press).

We have integrated both of these principal ideas in a decision tree (see Figure 6.8). Reading research reveals that the caesura between initial and advanced reading encompasses approximately the first year in learning to read (at least in the Dutch language; Kappers, 1986; Licht, 1988; Licht, Bakker, Kok, & Bouma, 1988). The mean reading level at the end of grade 1 is fairly constant. It is (in Dutch) a phase during which most children have made automatic the initial skills in reading, at the same time as their reading strategy becomes more lingual (Kappers, 1986).

For most cases the decision tree can be used to determine which cerebral hemisphere should be stimulated. Generally, a clinician will determine the problem, considering both neuropsychological theories, and the phase at which the problems arose in learning to read. When more than one problem is found, therapy will start with the problem that is oldest developmentally.

Sometimes more information is needed to decide which hemisphere should be stimulated. These children present with suspected neurological dysfunction or lesions and may require further neuropsychological or even neurologic examinations before proceeding with treatment. These complementary data can help determine whether specific stimulation of a hemisphere would be of practical benefit. If it is not clear whether the hemisphere in which a dysfunction or lesion is found could profit from specific stimulation, remedial treatment of the hemisphere can be started and closely monitored. If the remedial treatment fails to produce adequate benefits according to advanced formulated criteria, compensating treatment of the "intact" hemisphere should be initiated.

Case 1: Alice

Intake

At intake Alice was 11 years of age and had been attending a special-education school for two years as a result of her reading and spelling problems. Prior to that school, Alice had been attending regular classes. Her WISC-RN total IQ was average (TIQ = 96) with a significiant discrepancy between verbal and performance IQ (VIQ = 86, PIQ = 109). Her mother reported that she herself was a slow reader and that a brother of Alice's father had also been dyslexic.

Even though she had already received more than five years of reading instruction, including special help, her reading was halfway through grade 3, a discrepancy of two and a half years.

Alice made time-consuming (fragmentations) and substantive errors and her reading style was uncertain as well as slovenly. She repeated words unnecessarily and made guessing errors (words that were visually similar) and errors in the grapheme-phoneme translation.

Although her reading was on the advanced level, we found indications of possible nonoptimal mediation by the right cerebral hemisphere as well as the left. Therefore, according to the decision tree (Figure 6.8), we started with stimulation of the right cerebral hemisphere. Goals for treatment were (1) general increase in reading level, and (2) more accurate reading style. After reaching the first two goals, we would aim for (3) a more fluent reading style.

Treatment and Results

Alice's treatment was conducted in seven phases consisting of eight weekly treatment sessions of 50 minutes each. The period of treatment was just over one year.

During the first five treatment phases the right hemisphere was stimulated. In the first phase a tactile training box was used. On a planning board within the training box was fixed a piece of text at an appropriate instructional level. Alice was then asked to read the text by touch, using her left hand. During this task the child could hear her own voice, and that of the therapist, via her left ear while instrumental music was played to the right ear. All was accomplished by means of special headphones and an amplifier especially constructed for this purpose. In addition to these treatments, flash cards were used to strengthen automatizing of the grapheme-phoneme connection. These cards were given throughout the first five treatment phases. As appears in Figure 6.9, the first phase in treatment increased both word and text reading. Alice's reading was both faster and more accurate.

In the second phase, a visual half-field stimulation method was added to the treatment program. The RH was stimulated by means of the HEMSTIM program. Alice was asked to read aloud words that were

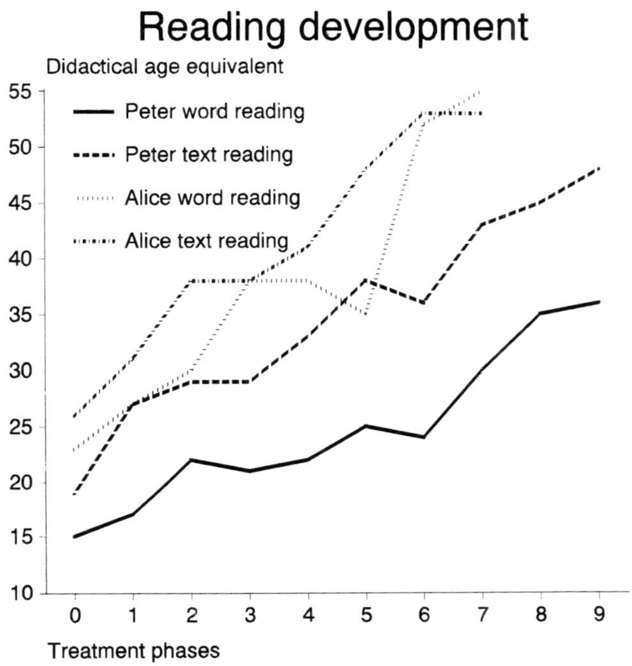

Fig. 6.9. The results of neuropsychological treatment on word and text reading of Alice and Peter.

flashed in the left visual field. Also during this excercise the special amplifier and headphones were again used for additional auditory stimulation. Although reading levels showed another increase (see Figure 6.9), Alice's reading style remained slovenly when faced with difficult pieces of text.

In the third phase, tactile training was replaced with an audio recording of short fragments of Alice's reading for use in self-correction. This phase of treatment further increased word reading by lessening errors and repetitions, but text reading showed no further increase. When reading text Alice was less accurate than when reading words, although she more often corrected her errors.

From results thus far, it appeared that context was difficult for Alice and so she was given homework in the fourth and fifth phase to work on this problem. Each week, in addition to the training program outlined in the third phase, Alice was given five pages of text for homework, and was asked to read one page each day. Although the text was at a suitable instructional level, it was printed in a perceptually demanding format (see Figure 6.7) to add a right-hemisphere alluding stimulation to the treatment program. Unlike word reading, text reading increased in the fourth and fifth phases.

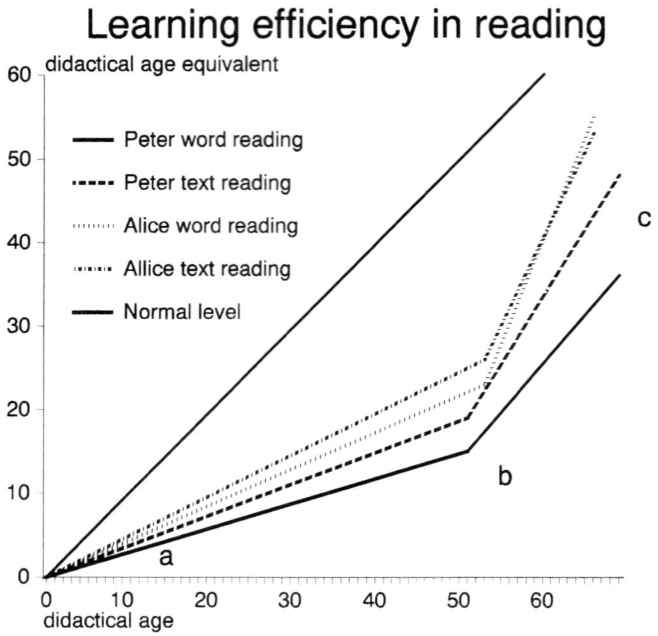

Fig. 6.10. Survey of the reading developments of Alice and Peter; a–b is the preintervention line, b the start of the intervention, and b–c the intervention line.

At the end of the fifth phase, it was concluded that the grapheme-phoneme connections were automatic and that reading style was accurate enough (and reading ability was sufficiently advanced) to switch treatment to stimulating the left cerebral hemisphere. The latter was accomplished in the sixth and seventh phases of treatment by using the visual half-field method. Words were now presented in the right visual field and had to be read aloud or monitored to detect specific sounds within the words. The tape-recording exercise was continued also. In both exercises all verbal information was presented to the right ear and instrumental music was presented to the left ear.

Treatment was terminated after the seventh phase because it was concluded that (1) her reading level was appropriate for her grade level (see Figure 6.9), (2) her reading style was relatively fluent and accurate, and (3) text comprehension was at a level appropriate for her grade.

For Alice, treatment resulted in a 2½-year catch-up in reading ability over about 13 months. Her learning efficiency in reading, which was 43 to 49% before treatment, increased to 246% for reading words and 207% for reading text after treatment (see Figure 6.10).

Case 2: Peter

Peter was twelve and had been enrolled in a school for special education for three years at the time of intake. Before being enrolled in that school Peter had twice attempted grade 1 in an elementary school. His intelligence was average (WISC-RN TIQ = 100), but a significant discrepancy was found between his verbal IQ (86) and his performance IQ (118).

His EEG showed a focal irritative disturbance in the left temporal lobe with a possible extension to the frontal lobe having hypofunctional character.

At age six, drains were placed in his eardrum because of recurrent inflammation in the middle ear.

Onset of speech was normal but development was not optimal and speech therapy was necessary. Despite receiving five years of remedial reading instruction, Peter's single-word reading was at a level midway through grade 2 and his text reading was at a level toward the end of grade 2. Therefore his reading discrepancy was 3 to 3½ years. Although his reading style was very accurate, he made many repetitions even when there was no motive to do so. His knowledge of grapheme-phoneme connections was not sufficiently automatic.

Treatment and Results

The goals for treatment were: (1) Automation of the weak subskill, (2) increasing speed and level of reading and, in a later phase, (3) concentration on a more fluent reading style.

Peter's treatment was conducted in nine phases and consisted of weekly treatments of 50 minutes each, except in the first phase. Each of the nine phases took two months to complete and duration of treatment was eighteen months.

In the first treatment phase Peter was trained at home by his parents for eight minutes a day. Flash cards were used to automatize the grapheme-phoneme connections and this simple training resulted in an a two-month increase in word reading and an eight-month increase in text reading (see Figure 6.9).

Although he had mastered the grapheme-phoneme connections it was decided that to maintain this mastery and to reach a stage of "over-learning," the flash-card exercise would be continued.

Because he was now an accurate reader and had mastered the subskills but still made too many tc errors (fragmentations; slow reading), it was decided that stimulation of the left cerebral hemisphere (see Figure 6.8) should continue throughout the treatment program.

In phase 2, the exercise with flash cards was continued during the treatment sessions. The main part of the treatment consisted of specific stimulation of the left cerebral hemisphere with the tactile training box, the amplifier, and the earphones as described before. At the end of phase 2, an additional five-month increase was seen in the level of word reading and a two-month increase was seen in text reading.

In phase 3, a five-minute reading-aloud exercise was taped and Peter was later asked to correct his reading. Following this phase of treatment, no increase was observed in text reading level and a slight decrease in word reading was seen (see Figure 6.9).

In phase 4, the reading-aloud and correcting exercise was replaced by words flashed in the right visual half-field using the Hemstim-program in combination with the auditory-stimulation technique described previously. This treatment phase increased text reading, mainly because of greater reading speed and recovery of the slight decrease in word reading.

From phase 5 on, the treatment program concentrated on fluency in reading. The treatment consisted of specific stimulation of the left cerebral hemisphere by the visual half-field technique described before. The reading-aloud and correction excercise was also reintroduced. The results of this treatment, phases 5 through 9, can be seen in Figure 6.9.

Over the entire treatment period Peter increased his text reading ability by nearly three years. During treatment his learning efficiency increased from 37% (preintervention) to 160% (see Figure 6.10). Peter had become a faster and more fluent reader. His text comprehension exceeded his text reading level by six months and his single-word reading had increased by two years: a learning efficiency of 117% compared to 29% in the pre-intervention period (see Figure 6.10).

Conclusion

The two case studies show that it is possible to reinitiate a long-stagnating learning-to-read process by applying the neuropsychological treatment procedures described in this chapter. We do not mean to say, however, that success can be anticipated in all cases of dyslexia. Clearly, questions still need to be answered, including how to integrate neuropsychological and nonneuropsychological methods of treatment.

Conclusion

According to the Balance Model, initial and advanced stages in the learning-to-read process are predominantly subserved by the right and the left cerebral hemispheres, respectively. Neuropsychological and electrophysiological evidence has been found supporting this model. Dyslexia may result if failure affects the shift in hemispheric mediation of reading at an appropriate stage in learning to read. Children who fail to make this shift become stuck in the early reading strategies generated by the right hemisphere (P-type dyslexia), whereas children who make the shift too early begin using left-hemisphere strategies prematurely (L-type dyslexia). Research into the validity of the P/L classification system has determined that cognitive and attentional parameters, as well as some of their electrophysiological correlates, differentiated between P and L types of dyslexia. Neuropsychological treatment is chosen as the next step in managing dyslexia on the assumption that the brain is sensitive to stimulation from the learning environment. Thus one would predict that stimulating the left hemisphere in P dyslexics and the right hemisphere in L dyslexics would change the lateral distribution of brain activity. In experimental research on subtype-X treatment interaction such changes were observed and were found to be correlated with specific improvements in reading. Neuropsychological treatment of dyslexia by specific or alluding stimulation is currently a facility in some child psychiatric/neurologic outpatient clinics and classroom learning centers.

The Balance Model of learning to read and dyslexia is compatible with the Novelty Model of hemispheric differences in acquiring and using of descriptive systems. The P/L classification of dyslexia, as arising from the Balance Model, shows similarities with other typologies of learning disabilities.

The observed effects of hemisphere stimulation on the lateral distribution of brain activity and subprocesses in reading demonstrate how useful neuropsychological treatment procedures are. Similar procedures may prove to promote acquisition or reacquisition of other hemisphere-mediated functions. Applying any neuropsychological treatment, however, presupposes sufficient knowledge about the brain's systems and mechanisms that do now or eventually will subserve the functions that one wants to address therapeutically.

Acknowledgment. The authors thank Karen Eso, M.A., for her comments on English grammar and style.

References

Aro, M., Licht, R., & Lyytinen, H. (1993). *Do probe ERP's reveal differences between the subtypes of developmental dyslexia?* Poster presented at the 3rd European Congress of Psychology, Tampere, Finland, July.

August, G.J., & Garfinkel, B.D. (1990). Comorbidity of ADHD and reading disability among clinically referred children. *Journal of Abnormal Psychology, 18,* 29–45.

Bakker, D.J. (1973). Hemispheric specialization and stages in the learning to read process. *Bulletin of the Orton Society, 23,* 15–27.

Bakker, D.J. (1979a). Hemispheric differences and reading strategies: Two dyslexias? *Bulletin of the Orton Society, 29,* 84–100.

Bakker, D.J. (1979b). Perceptual asymmetries and reading proficiency. In M. Bortner (Ed.), *Cognitive growth and development* (pp. 134–152). New York: Brunner/Mazel.

Bakker, D.J. (1980). Dyslexia in developmental neuropsychology: Hemisphere-specific models. In D.J. Oborne, M.M. Gruneberg, & J.R. Eiser (Eds.), *Psychology and Medicine* (pp. 347–353). London: Academic Press.

Bakker, D.J. (1986). *Zijdelings: Neuropsychologische methoden ter behandeling van dyslexieën*. Lisse, Netherlands: Swets & Zeitlinger.

Bakker, D.J. (1989). Boosting the (dyslexic) brain. In D.J. Bakker & H. van der Vlugt (Eds.), *Learning disabilities: Neuropsychological correlates and treatment* (pp. 173–181). Lisse, Netherlands: Swets & Zeitlinger.

Bakker, D.J. (1990). *Neuropsychological treatment of dyslexia*. New York: Oxford University Press.

Bakker, D.J. (1992). Neuropsychological classification and treatment of dyslexia. *Journal of Learning Disabilities, 25,* 102–109.

Bakker, D.J., Smink, T., & Reitsma, P. (1973). Ear dominance and reading ability. *Cortex, 9,* 301–312.

Bakker, D.J., Moerland, M.C., & Goekoop-Hoefkens, M. (1981). Effects of hemisphere-specific stimulation on the reading performance of dyslexic boys: A pilot study. *Journal of Clinical Neuropsychology, 3,* 155–159.

Bakker, D.J., & Vinke, J. (1985). Effects of hemisphere-specific stimulation on brain activity and reading in dyslexics. *Journal of Clinical and Experimental Neuropsychology, 7,* 505–525.

Bakker, D.J., Bouma, A., & Gardien, C.J. (1990). Hemisphere-specific treatment of dyslexia subtypes: A field experiment. *Journal of Learning Disabilities, 23,* 433–438.

Bakker, M.G., Spyer, G., & Hoekman, P. (1990). Hemisphere-alluding stimulation as a catalyst in the HSS-treatment of L-dyslexia. *Journal of Clinical and Experimental Neuropsychology, 12,* 196.

Bakker, D.J., Licht, R., & Van Strien, J. (1991). Biopsychological validation of L- and P-type dyslexia. In B.P. Rourke (Ed.), *Neuropsychological validation of learning disability subtypes* (pp. 124–139). New York: Guilford Press.

Barron, R.W. (1986). Word recognition in early reading: A review of the direct and indirect access hypotheses. *Cognition, 24,* 93–119.

Boder, E. (1973). Developmental dyslexia: A diagnostic approach based on three atypical reading-spelling patterns. *Developmental Medicine and Child Neurology, 15,* 663–687.

Bos, M., & Van Vliet, M. (1990). *P-of-L type: Normen voor het indelen van dyslectische kinderen die lezen op AVI-niveau een of twee*. Unpublished Master's Thesis, Free University, Amsterdam, Netherlands.

Carmon, A., Nachshon, I., & Starinsky, R. (1976). Developmental aspects of visual hemifield differences in perception of verbal material. *Brain and Language, 3,* 463–469.

De Sonneville, L.M.J. (1993). SVAT: A computer-based approach to development and disorders of information processing. In F.J. Maarse, A.E. Akkerman, N. Brand, L.J.M. Mulder, & M. Van der Stelt (Eds.), *Computers in psychology, Vol. 4* (pp. 168–176). Lisse, Netherlands: Swets & Zeitlinger.

De Sonneville, L.M.J., Neijens, L., & Licht, R. (1993). Leer-en aandachtsstoornissen: Vroegtijdige onderkenning en samenhang. In E.J.M. Van Aarle & K. Henneman (Eds.), *Dyslexie 1992* (pp. 17–27). Lisse, Netherlands: Swets & Zeitlinger.

Dumont, J.J. (1990). *Dyslexie: Theorie, diagnostiek, behandeling*. Rotterdam: Lemniscaat.

De Sonneville, L.M.J., Leek, M., & Licht, R. (in preparation). Aandachts-skoornissen bij twee typen dyslectische kinderen.

Dykman, R.A., & Ackerman, P.T. (1991). Attention deficit disorder and specific reading disability: Separate but often overlapping disorders. *Journal of Learning Disabilities, 19,* 426–431.

Fletcher, J.M., & Morris, R. (1986). Classification of disabled readers: Beyond exclusionary definitions. In C.J. Ceci (Ed.), *Handbook of cognitive, social, and neuropsychological aspects of learning disabilities, Vol. I* (pp. 55–80). Hillsdale, NJ: Lawrence Erlbaum.

Frederiksen, J.R. (1980). Component skills in reading: Measurement of in dividual differences through chronometric analysis. In R.E. Snow, P.A. Federico, & W.E. Montague (Eds.), *Aptitude, learning and instruction, Vol. I* (pp. 105–138). Hillsdale, NJ: Lawrence Erlbaum.

Fries, C.C. (1963). *Linguistics and reading.* New York: Holt, Rinehart & Winston.

Goldberg, E., & Costa, L.D. (1981). Hemispheric differences in the acquisition and use of descriptive systems. *Brain and Language, 14,* 144–173.

Grace, G.M., & Spreen, O. (in press). Hemisphere-specific stimulation of L and P types: A replication study and a critical appraisal. In R. Licht & G. Spyer (Eds.), *Bakker's balance model of dyslexia.* Lisse, Netherlands: Swets & Zeitlinger.

Harter, M.R., & Aine, C.J. (1984). Brain mechanism of visual selective attention. In R. Parasuraman & D.R. Davies (Eds.), *Varieties of attention* (pp. 293–321). New York: Academic Press.

Heilman, K.M., & Van den Abell, T. (1979). Right hemispheric dominance for mediating cerebral activation. *Neuropsychologia, 17,* 315–321.

Hillyard, S.A. (1984). Event-related potentials and selective attention. In E. Donchin (Ed.), *Cognitive psychophysiology: Event-related potentials and the study of cognition* (pp. 51–72). Hillsdale, NJ: Lawrence Erlbaum.

Hooper, S.R., & Willis, W.G. (1989). *Learning disability subtyping.* New York: Springer-Verlag.

Jonkman, I., Licht, R., Bakker, D.J., & Van den Broek-Sandmann, T.M. (1992). Shifting of attention in subtyped dyslexic children: An event-related potential study. *Developmental Neuropsychology, 8,* 243–259.

Kappers, E.J. (1986). *Structureringstendentie, hemisfeerspecialisatie en leren lezen.* Unpublished Doctoral Dissertation, State University, Utrecht.

Kappers, E.J. (1993). Een opmaat naar zorg op maat: Van theoriën naar be-handeling van ernstige leesproblemen. In H.M. Pijnenburg & L.M.G. Curfs (Eds.), *Jaarboek onderzoek pedologische instituten 1992.* Cadier en Keer: Lopi.

Kappers, E.J., & Hamburger, H.L. (in press). Neuropsychological treatment of dyslexia in out-patients. In R. Licht & G. Spyer (Eds.), *Bakker's balance model of dyslexia.* Lisse, Netherlends: Swets & Zeitlinger.

Leek, M. (1993). *Aandachts-controle bij dyslectische kinderen.* Unpublished Master's Thesis, Free University, Amsterdam.

Licht, R. (1988). *Event-related potential asymmetries and word reading in children: A developmental study.* Unpublished Doctoral Dissertation, Free University, Amsterdam.

Licht, R. (1989). Reading disability subtypes: Cognitive and electrophysiological differences. In D.J. Bakker & H. v.d. Vlugt (Eds.), *Learning disabilities* (Vol. 1, pp. 81–103). Lisse, Netherlands: Swets & Zeitlinger.

Licht, R. (in press). Differences in components of word recognition between P- and L-type reading disability. In R.M. Joshi & C.K. Leong (Eds.), *Developmental and acquired dyslexia: Neuropsychological and neurolinguistic perspectives*. Kluwer Academic Publishers.

Licht, R., Bakker, D.J., Kok, A., & Bouma, A. (1988). The development of lateral event-related potentials (ERP's) related to word naming: A 4-year longitudinal study. *Neuropsychologia, 26,* 327–340.

Licht, R., Jonkman, I., Bakker, D.J., & Woestenburg, J. (1990). Selective attention and hemispheric asymmetry in two dyslexia subtypes: An electrophysiological (ERP) approach. In W. Koops & H. Soppe (Eds.), *Developmental psychology behind the dykes* (pp. 181–192). Delft, Netherlands: Eburon.

Mitterer, J.O. (1982). There are at least two kinds of poor readers: Whole word readers and recoding poor readers. *Canadian Journal of Psychology, 36,* 445–461.

Moerland, M.C., & Bakker, D.J. (1993). Hemstim 1.0: A computerized treatment program for children suffering from P-type or L-type dyslexia. In F.J. Maarse, A.E. Akkerman, A.N. Brand, L.J.M. Mulder, & J.J. van der Stelt (Eds.), *Computers in psychology: Tools for experimental and applied psychology* (pp. 151–158). Lisse, Netherlands: Swets & Zeitlinger.

Neijens, L. (1991). *Betrouwbaarheid en validiteit van classificatie in type dyslexie volgens het balansmodel.* Unpublished Master's Thesis, Catholic University Brabant, Tilbung.

Neuvonen, M., Rekio-Viinikainen, N., Ahonen, T., & Lyytinen, H. (1992). Tietokoneelle sovellettu Bakkerin tasapainomalliin perustuva lukemisen kuntoutus. *Kielikukko, 4,* 26–29.

Pirozzolo, F.J. (1979). *The neuropsychology of developmental reading disorders.* New York: Praeger Press.

Posner, M.I. (1978). *Chronometric explorations of mind.* Hillsdale, NJ: Lawrence Erlbaum Associates.

Renner, M.J., & Rosenzweig, M.R. (1987). *Enriched and impoverished environments: Effects on brain and behavior.* New York: Springer-Verlag.

Rourke, B.P. (1982). Central processing deficiencies in children: Towards a developmental neuropsychological model. *Journal of Clinical Neuropsychology, 4,* 1–18.

Rourke, B.P., & Petrauskas, R.J. (1977). Underlining test (Revised). Windsor, Ontario: Authors.

Russo, A.E. (1993). *Effects of the presence of pathological left-handedness indicators on the efficacy of a neuropsychological intervention with low achieving readers.* Unpublished Doctoral Dissertation, University of Pennsylvania, Harrisburg.

Sadick, T.L., & Ginsburg, B.E. (1978). The development of the lateral functions and reading ability. *Cortex, 14,* 3–11.

Satz, P., & Morris, R. (1981). Learning disabilities subtypes: A review. In F.J. Pirozzolo & M.C. Wittrock (Eds.), *Neuropsychological and cognitive processes in reading* (pp. 109–141). New York: Academic Press.

Sternberg, S. (1969). Discovery of processing stages: Extensions of Donders' method. In W.G. Koster (Ed.), *Attention and Performance II* (pp. 276–315). Amsterdam: North-Holland.

Van Strien, J.W., Bakker, D.J., Bouma, A., & Koops, W. (1988). Familial antecedents of P- and L-type dyslexia. *Journal of Clinical and Experimental Neuropsychology*, *10*, 323.

Van Strien, J.W., Bouma, A., & Bakker, D.J. (1993). Lexical decision performances in P-type dyslexic, L-type dyslexic, and normal reading boys. *Journal of Clinical and Experimental Neuropsychology, 14,* 4, 516–524.

Van Strien, J.W., & Morpurgo, M. (1992). Opposite hemispheric activations as a result of emotionally threatening and nonthreatening words. *Neuropsychologia, 30,* 845–848.

Van Strien, J.W., Stolk, B., & Zuiker, S. (in press). Hemisphere-speific treatment of dyslexia subtypes: Better reading with threatening words? *Journal of Learning Disabilities*.

Verhulst, F.C., Koot, J.M., Akkerhuis, G.W., & Veerman, J.W. (1990). *Praktische handleiding voor de CBCL*. Assen, Netherlands: Van Gorcum.

Epilogue

Michael G. Tramontana and Stephen R. Hooper

This volume has continued with the tradition laid down in the two preceding volumes in this series. As before, each of the topics was dealt with in a rigorous and integrative manner. There were further examples of innovative work and "cutting-edge" research, with new data presented in a number of cases. Practical linkages were drawn where appropriate, and key questions were raised for each advance or fresh insight put forth. All of this was in keeping with the aims of the *Advances* series.

Chapter 1, by Dennis L. Molfese, provided an extension of the longitudinal work initially presented in Volume 1 of this series—this time, with a larger group of children and a more complex array of variables examined. This was an unusual opportunity to follow an important and exciting line of developmental investigation as it unfolds. Again, an impressive case was made for the utility of auditory evoked responses obtained in early infancy in predicting subsequent cognitive and language development during the preschool years.

In the following section, David Bellinger (Chapter 2) gave us a thoughtful discussion on the neurotoxic effects of lead, focusing especially on the well-known Boston Prospective Study. This has been a controversial area of inquiry, in which research findings and public policy guidelines continue to be hotly debated. Yet, more is known about lead than any other toxin to date. Bellinger's chapter not only details this, but also presents the many complexities involved in forming valid inferences regarding neurodevelopmental effects. In doing this, it provides a prototypic set of questions that should guide investigations dealing with other neurotoxins.

Next, a cluster of chapters dealt with complementary aspects of assessment. One by Erin D. Bigler (Chapter 3) illustrated major advances in brain imaging techniques. These exciting developments should have an unprecedented impact on the advancement of knowledge in child neuropsychology, especially concerning the neural side of brain–behavior relationships. Progress, however, will also depend on parallel advances in conceptualizing and assessing the behavioral aspects of these relationships through the development of more precise and ecologically valid tools for assessing neuropsychological functioning. This was covered from two perspectives: Marit Korkman's presentation (Chapter 4) on the development and rationale behind the NEPSY, a novel approach to child neuropsychological assessment; and Antonia A. Forster and Ingrid N. Leckliter's presentation (Chapter 5), which focused instead on advances in the construct validation of existing methods, especially as they relate to the evaluation of working memory.

Recruiting contributions dealing with exemplary work in the area of treatment has been one of the more challenging aspects of editing this series. As noted previously, work that bridges that gap between assessment and treatment continues to represent a relatively undeveloped territory in child neuropsychology. Interventions with a strong foundation of empirical validation are even rarer. In this context, the work of Dirk J. Bakker, Robert Licht, and E. Jan Kappers (Chapter 6) on hemispheric stimulation methods in dyslexia is truly remarkable. There is hardly a better example in child neuropsychology of a paradigmatic line of investigation linking assessment and treatment that is both theory driven and empirically validated—a rare find indeed.

Overall, as with the preceding volumes, Volume 3 has provided yet another glimpse of the ever-expanding knowledge and exciting developments unfolding in the field of child neuropsychology. Once again, we consider ourselves most fortunate to have assembled an international cast of contributors sharing their important findings, insights, and thoughtful questions. We are extremely pleased in how they have helped us to embrace the spirit and objectives that we set out to meet with *Advances in Child Neuropsychology*.

Index

E

F

G

H

I

K

L

P

Q

R

S

T

U

V

W